Rock And Roll At Any Age

A rebellious look at life, health, and spiritual wisdom from the "Sassy Sage"

By Joan Lubar

Dear Pat,
What a pleasure
to meet you! To the
best of success & joy as
you Rock + Roll into the future!
fondly,
Joan

Love Your Life

Wilmington, Delaware

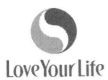

Love Your Life Publishing

Wilmington, DE

www.loveyourlifepublishing.com

ISBN: 978-1-934509-91-3

Library of Congress Control Number: 2016963467

Printed in the United States of America

First Printing

Editing by Gwen Hoffnagle

CONTENTS

FOREWORD

I've been on a quest to find the eternal fountain of youth for years... actually decades. I've read dozens of books, hundreds of magazine articles, listened to podcast shows, been to workshops and seminars, and tried just about every diet known to mankind (and womankind). I search for answers.

When I first met Joan Lubar many years ago at a workshop I hosted in Portland, Oregon, I was struck by her vibrancy and energy. Out of nearly one hundred people in the room, Joan's energy was infectious. She played full out, made others laugh with her spirited sense of humor, and made it obvious she was willing to do whatever it took to get the most out of the experience.

When she shared her age with the group, there was a palatable gasp from the other women in the room. Joan defied the odds of what it meant to be an older woman. She had more spunk and energy than women half her age.

Her "can do" attitude was one I was curious about; obviously she had not experienced many obstacles in her life. Yet when she shared what drives her, I discovered that not only has she encountered incredibly difficult times in her life, she has managed to transcend the toughest times while maintaining a very positive attitude.

What was her secret? I wanted to know. As I got to know Joan, I discovered a woman who has been on a quest to learn as much about living a healthy, vibrant, and passionate life as she could for the better part of forty years—one in which she has made it her life's work to understand health and nutrition in a way that is rarely found these days.

I also learned more about what gives Joan the type of energy and passion she has. It's a result of what she eats, the types of supplements she takes, and an attitude that we can get through anything and live with grace if we choose to.

In *Rock and Roll at Any Age,* Joan freely shares insights into her life that will make you eager to learn as much as you can from this amazing woman. Each chapter is filled with sage wisdom Joan has applied to her own life for decades—wisdom that helps her clients improve their own health.

As I discovered how dedicated to the well-being of others Joan truly is, I incorporated a new protocol of supplements into my own daily regime as well as many of the ways of eating Joan recommends. As a woman in my sixties, I feel better than I thought possible. I have more than enough energy to participate in a sport I took up when I turned sixty-one... running.

The more I get to know Joan, the more I realize what it means to live one's purpose. I now have the privilege and honor to call Joan a dear friend, a friend I know will defy the odds of aging more every day.

I can promise you this: By the time you finish *Rock and Roll at Any Age* you will have a completely renewed sense of what is possible with your health, your energy, and you attitude. In a society accustomed to hiding and disregarding our elders, Joan refuses to be quiet. She is on a mission to influence the lives of as many people as possible to live with vitality and vibrancy and not be hidden away and disregarded.

Joan is one who definitely lives the role of the Sassy Sage. *Rock and Roll at Any Age* is a must-read for anyone who is not willing to settle for the status quo or be at the mercy of our healthcare system. In this rebellious look at life, health, and spiritual wisdom, Joan will leave you laughing, crying, and thanking your lucky stars you have in your hands one of the best books on living your life on purpose that you've read in a long, long time.

Kathleen Gage
Author, speaker, and late-in-life runner
www.passionforthriving.com

INTRODUCTION

When I was young, many different people and attitudes influenced how I thought about myself and what I believed about culture, religion, and health. Some of my more engrained beliefs were around aging—what getting old looked like, how I fed and moved my body, how older women and men became disregarded and marginalized.

As I've aged, I've realized that many of those beliefs no longer serve me. I began to shed what no longer made sense. As it does for all of us, life took me through years of emotional, physical, and spiritual challenges, and I engaged in some rigorous "unlearning" and "relearning." I questioned and examined—and opened up to new ways of thinking and new ways of seeing the world, my role, and my life.

At age forty, I was sick, heavy, and so exhausted I couldn't keep my eyes open at work. Now, at seventy-plus years old, I'm fit and fabulous. I'm ready for what's next. I'm healthy, slender, and have more energy than many who are half my age. I wake up excited to do what I love and serve more people. I'm a grandma who ballroom dances and does yoga and enjoys a beautiful community of people both younger and older than I am. I know I am a positive contribution to the people around me. I believe that there's much more that is possible in my life, and I still have a long list of dreams I want to achieve.

I have completely unlearned and relearned what it means to be an elder.

So why can't everyone feel this way? I wrote *Rock and Roll at Any Age* because I believe that everyone can. I believe that no matter what your state of health today, improvement can be yours. Vitality can be yours. Purpose and meaning can be yours. It takes a strong commitment to accept total responsibility for your health, but it's not as difficult as you might think.

In this book I share my stories so you can see how I got where I am today. I am no different from you; I simply made a decision thirty-four years ago to start changing my life and I have evolved to the fit and fabulous way I feel today.

Why did I call this book *Rock and Roll at Any Age*? Rock-and-rock has been the backdrop for my whole life, as it probably has been for yours. I was born the same year as Paul McCartney. I had just entered my teen years when rock-and-roll became popular, and as someone who loves to dance, I couldn't help but move my body. Since those early days of twisting and swinging my friends at the school dances, for me rock-and-roll has been the symbol of freedom, rebelliousness, and energy.

And now here we are. All we early rock-and-roll lovers are entering our senior years. As we age, many of us start thinking we have to act a certain way, dress a certain way, and behave "appropriately," whatever that means. That is where we go wrong. That is when we start to live in a limited way and miss so much of the richness our elder years can hold.

I say why not be rebellious? Why not age in a way no one expects? Why not keep moving and dancing and feeling free? The thing is, in order to do this, you have to feel great. You have to be healthy. I wrote this book to show you how.

OK?

Let's rock!

* * *

Please remember that these are my opinions, based on my life experiences and beliefs that have evolved over more than seventy years. These are the principles, attitudes, and products that have worked for me. People often tell me that I seem to have a glow on my face, a joy in life, and look at the cup as half full rather than half empty. They say, "You should write a book and show people how you do that." This book is simply my account of how I do that.

CHAPTER 1

HOW I BECAME THE SASSY SAGE

"Hot Stuff"

'Cause music is what I want
To keep my body always moving
Yeah, shake it up, hot stuff.

— The Rolling Stones

I feel eyes on me as I walk into the restaurant. I'm thirty-eight and wearing the amazing bright-yellow, strapless linen dress I just bought. I'm traveling with my two boys to Brazil's Iguacu Falls, one of the wonders of the world, and tonight we're going out to dinner. I have never felt more beautiful, even *sexy*, as we walk into the dining room. Thanks to working out three times at a week at a Brazilian spa, I'm slender and strong. My tan skin glows. I feel alive. Young. Empowered. What could be better?

Truth be told, *lots* could be better. Even though I feel beautiful and strong at this particular moment, my life is in shambles. My two boys are visiting from boarding school in the US as I'm struggling to end a very difficult marriage to their stepfather and move back home to the States. This mini-vacation with my sons is a way to escape the tensions in my unhappy Sao Paulo home. There is no peace of mind there, only hostility from a man who wants me to give up my children to stay with him. There is no way that will happen!

I'm a mess. I feel betrayed by his treatment of my boys and anxious that I can't easily leave Brazil. I wonder how I'll be able to support myself and my children when I return. I'm terrified and I have no one at home or in Brazil to talk to, no wise elder to give me sage advice and support. Calls back to my mom in the States are brief and not usually private.

I face all of this alone, filled with a potent mix of fear, stress, and resentment, holding myself together like a torn and tattered book patched with Scotch tape. Our trip to these magnificent falls is a brief and needed moment of joy before I step back into the thick tension at home.

When I recently told a friend how I felt that night more than thirty years ago, I said, "That night I felt the most exhilarated I had in a long time... And now, I have to tell you, I feel that way again."

It's true. I am in my seventies. And I feel exhilarated, empowered, and beautiful. But this beauty is not only on the surface as it was that day in Brazil. It's an internal, peaceful beauty that encompasses all of the lessons I have learned and my own tremendous personal growth from them. Today I feel strong and slender. My skin glows. And I am happy to report that I also feel focused, calm, and purposeful. My days have meaning. My life has meaning. These really are the best years of my life. Really!

I allowed those deep, dark days to become powerful lessons that helped me evolve mentally, emotionally, physically, and spiritually and follow the meaningful journey that I now share. As I listen to others' stories, I realize that my experience and the wisdom I've gleaned from it can provide some new perspective and ideas that help. I have been there — filled with fear, not knowing what the future holds, drained of confidence, wondering who I am.

These days friends and colleagues call me the "Sassy Sage" for a few reasons: Because I love to tease and see the humor in the dramas we create. Because they come to me for my listening ear and, hopefully, my sage advice. And because at age seventy-four, I look and feel at least a decade younger — and they want to know how I do it.

I wrote *Rock and Roll at Any Age* to share what I believe keeps me young and on top of my game, but I also have another motive up my sleeve. As good as I feel and as vibrant as I know I am, I also live in a culture that disregards and tosses out the very experience and wisdom that I can offer. Our throwaway society believes that power and brilliance belong to the young, and that they have the knowledge and energy to do it bigger and better. Our elders, once honored and respected and looked to for guidance in the storms of youth, are now hidden away and disregarded.

It's no secret that our world has run amok and many people are living hollow lives that lack meaning and purpose. I believe we need our wise ones back to show the way — to bring us all back to ourselves. The wisdom I've culled from my myriad experiences brings into sharp focus the need for me—and every one of us in our later years—to offer younger generations the wisdom and perspective they so desperately need. From there they can make decisions from a broader view, whether or not they agree with us.

Instead, however, we are hiding away our elders. Nursing homes and retirement homes are hugely profitable for the corporations that own them. Visits with our older relatives are more like dreaded, dutiful have-tos than they are warm, supportive exchanges. How did we get to this place? I have a theory. In the 1940s and '50s my parents and others like them doted on their children. They were thankful that we had come out of World War II whole. Those were the beginning years of prosperity and of the US becoming a world power. They wanted us to have it all, and provided as much of that—from bikes and dance lessons to white-picket-fence neighborhoods and college educations—as they could.

While these years were good ones, what unfolded in the decades that followed was tough to witness. I saw adults my age with materialistic attitudes coupled with arrogant assumptions that we were better than everyone else. We all assumed that this trend of growth and prosperity would just keep growing forever. My peers began to distance themselves from their parents, believing their new and better ideas didn't need the old folks' worn-out contributions. For many, the commitment to family that drove their parents was absent.

Then I watched as my peers' children took on these attitudes of disregard and disrespect, and in turn often rejected their elders without any attempt to listen to what they had to offer. There is a normal and natural balance-shifting that occurs between parent and child as the child grows up. Think of Cat Stevens's song "Father and Son" from the 1970s. That's not what I'm talking about. What we missed in my generation was the elders transmitting their *wisdom*. And when this happened, we lost out on all they built; their sense of community and family; and the blood, sweat, and tears they shed in order to provide for those close to them.

It is a tragic loss. When I see nursing homes filled with old folks who've been abandoned, undernourished, and resigned to wheelchairs, it is beyond heartbreaking. This is not what's meant to happen! And not only is this putting our youth at risk by making them more fearful and rudderless without the guidance of those who've gone before, it's disorienting for elders, too.

The traditional role of elders included remembering what was most important about life and how to hold ends and beginnings together when times become hard. Being "old enough to know better," they would know that life renews itself in surprising ways and that the greatest dilemmas can serve to awaken the deepest resources of the human soul.

– *Michael Meade,* Why the World Doesn't End

It is time to help our younger folks realize that elders offer ways of thinking and mentoring that can guide younger folks through difficult and perplexing times. That they can savor and assess all the different outlooks that come from our successes and missteps. That the journeys elders have been through not only matter, they are also vital to the world and to the next generations. That they can trust themselves to follow their natural instincts to turn to the older folks when things get hard. This does not imply they should do what older folks say. Not at all. Having the seasoned perspective, however, can allow for more knowledgeable decisions.

And that, my friends, is part of my mission in writing *Rock and Roll at Any Age*. I want to help create a well-rounded community of all ages working together to achieve a better world. And I have met so many people interested in accomplishing this same BIG dream.

To do this, however, those of us in our sixties, seventies, and beyond must remain healthy, think and communicate clearly, and in many ways be able to keep up with the younger generations. We need to earn back that role that has slipped away. (Remember the rebelliousness of rock-and-roll that I was talking about?)

Just imagine what could be possible in your life if — every day — you felt invigorated, full of energy, and able to actively participate with those much younger? Imagine what could be possible for the world? I am not talking about discovering the fountain of youth or seventy-five-year-olds running marathons faster than thirty-year-olds. What I am talking about is thriving and creating a meaningful life by taking total responsibility for your own health and well-being.

I'm talking about people like me. I am in great shape physically and have energy to do more things than people half my age. (I often tire my kids out just by describing what I've done on a given day.) I love learning, sharing, and creating a better life. I choose to live in a world of fulfillment, not decay. I take responsibility for everything that happens to me in my life and every single choice I make. What if you could navigate your later years like this? (Believe me, the sooner you start, the better!)

For years now I have heard cries of despair from people who dread each birthday and fear what "aging" has in store for them. Are you one of them? Are you afraid that wrinkles will turn everyone against you? Do you imagine hobbling down the street sure that everyone is looking at you with pity? Perhaps you are positive you will end up with high blood pressure, a heart attack, or worse yet, Alzheimer's. How old were you when you started this descent into worry, self-pity, and fear?

For some, including me, it begins very young. I was forty when the doctor gave me the bad news: the discomfort I was feeling was fibroid tumors and I needed a hysterectomy. "When you are uncomfortable enough," my doctor said, "it will be time to remove them." I was soon uncomfortable enough.

With the knowledge I have today about how our bodies can naturally heal, perhaps I could have gotten rid of those pesky tumors without surgery, but instead I can now thank them, as they signaled the beginning of a new life for me.

I had the surgery — but I didn't bounce back afterwards. In fact, I was exhausted, falling asleep at work, and gaining weight. No one told me that after such a major assault on my physical body I'd need nutritional help to repair and rebuild me.

I have since also learned that for every emotional action there is a physical reaction. What I mean is that our physical bodies reveal what is going on inside our heads. That might be anything from having a feeling of embarrassment that results in blushing to having significant, prolonged stress develop into a major disease.

Illness, disease, and premature aging are not givens. They often result from a combination of several lifestyle and life events. I began to learn this in 1983 as I was recovering from that surgery. Like so many of us, my life was very full with work and children. Add two divorces and an ADHD child, and to say the least, I was under just a little stress. I had no idea that the emotional side of life could totally impact my physical health. I also had no idea that what I ate played such an important role in my health. As I write this I wonder how I could *not* have known — it seems so obvious today. But like so many, I was uneducated in some of the very basics of optimal living and health. I made a decision to change that and learn all I could about it.

I'm no different from you or anyone else. But as a woman in my seventies, having spent over thirty years intentionally creating my life as I want it to be, I look years younger, feel better, and enjoy life more than most. Many have asked me to share my story, the lessons I've learned, and strategies I've used to reach this age with so much vitality.

I am still sure I can't be any older than fifty, though that year is forced to rise every year as my oldest son's age advances! In fact, I prefer counting my age biologically and spiritually as opposed to chronologically. I agree with Dr. Christiane Northrup, who shares only her biological age and her "wisdom" age. As you can see from my picture, I am not your grandmother's seventy-four-year-old! No one has been able to guess my age correctly for years now. My new way of telling people my age is to say, "I'm biologically forty and my wisdom age is two hundred and fifty!"

For those of you entering that mysterious world of being a senior and wondering how to make the most of it, why not join me? And for those who are younger, what better time to begin this journey than right now? I promise you, what you do today will make all the difference in your forties, fifties, sixties, and beyond.

After all of these wisdom-gathering years, jam-packed with choices that worked well and not so well, here I am sharing my own strategies from lessons learned so that perhaps you, too, can age feeling full of pep, play with your grandchildren, and look at life as something that invigorates and fascinates on a daily basis. Eventually you can take your place as an *elder* in our society — instead of as someone who's just *older*.

I invite you to read on to learn how to nourish yourself, give back to your family and community, and help the younger generation move closer to lives of collaboration and connectedness. We all need it so much.

Your game is never over. Far from it. Imagine what kind of world this will be when your wisdom becomes a gift to be shared, and when you feel fantastic and healthy enough to want to share it!

Let's get started.

CHAPTER 2

KNOW WHERE YOU ARE TO GET WHERE YOU'RE GOING

"You Ain't Seen Nothing Yet"

You ain't seen nothin' yet
B-B-B-Baby, you just ain't seen nothin' yet
Here's something that you never gonna forget
B-B-B-Baby, you just ain't seen nothin' yet.

— *Bachman-Turner Overdrive*

Why are you really reading this book? I hope you picked it up because you want to live with a sense of fun, fulfillment, abandonment, and positive expectation for the future. And you want tips and strategies for making that happen.

Perhaps today you feel sluggish, you're not sleeping well, or have spotted some new wrinkles. Maybe you're panicking that life will never be the same again because old age is creeping in. Things might be really rough: You might be overweight, unhappy at work, or in a miserable relationship. Or maybe life is great—you're doing all the right things for your health and well-being and just want some new ideas and inspiration.

If you're young, congratulations for picking up this book. Believe me, the stresses of child-rearing and the culmination of choices you make when you're young affect your later years. Like a retirement account, starting early to build health shows up in your vibrancy twenty, thirty, and forty years down the road.

At my first yoga class, when I was in my twenties, I met a woman in her fifties. She had started yoga because her seventy-six-year-old aunt had begun a few years before and could now stand on her head! She wanted to do that, too. I realized in that moment that we truly can make changes at any age, successfully. So WELCOME, wherever you are!

These later years have been some of the best of my life. I feel lucky and grateful that I had a wonderful childhood with loving parents who made sure my days were filled with fun and interesting activities. I was fortunate. Still, as children, the world is centered around us—when we don't get what we want or are scolded for doing what feels natural to us, we experience frustration, disappointment, and wrongness. As children we can't always understand the emotional ups and downs we experience.

As we grow, navigating life circumstances can lead to feelings of self-doubt, poor self-esteem, and heartache. Even small hurts and casual criticisms can grow into self-doubt, anxiety, or anger. Instead of feeling like life is full of possibility and adventure, we start to feel "I can't," "I shouldn't," or

"I have to." We become afraid of failure and loss... and of disapproval. (How many things have you done or not done out of fear of the disapproval of others! Oy!)

This low-level anxiety and fear governs us. For many women—especially those over fifty—self-doubt and not-good-enough are such familiar feelings we don't even notice them anymore. That's certainly how it was for me when I was younger. Because of a thyroid condition, I experienced severe hair loss from the ages of thirteen to fifteen, and that took a toll on how I felt about myself, despite my parents' best intentions in helping me feel okay about it. As I grew older my doubts and fears and low self-esteem only grew.

Thankfully, part of getting older (ideally) is gaining the wisdom and understanding of our own humanity. This helps me accept those things I cannot change in my past or in somebody else's behavior. I accept that we all do the best we can do in each moment, even if it is not always the best we are capable of. Healing my old wounds and forgiving myself for when I feel I failed have helped me maintain a joyful attitude—no matter what happens—as I live with a sense of continued possibilities instead of fear, anxiety, and worry about disapproval.

My goal is that you will understand this and be able to create and nourish your own possibilities when you are finished reading this book.

Okay, first things first. Where are you now?

If you wanted to travel from your home to Fairbanks, Alaska, what would you need? At the very least, you'd need a map, a plan, and the desire to get there. But the very first thing you'd need is to know exactly where you are. Well, it's the same in your life.

If you don't know exactly where you are now, where you want to go, and why you want to get there, chances are you'll either never arrive or you'll get lost along the way. To begin this journey you have to look hard at yourself and understand all that brought you to this point.

My personal journey began in earnest after two failed marriages. I had to examine why I had made such bad choices and why I settled for two relationships that I knew deep inside were not right for me. When I started looking, here's what I found: Growing up female in the 1950s, I learned from my parents, especially my mother, that I was expected to go to college in order to have a degree to "fall back on" just in case, and ultimately get married and have kids. My mother always regretted that she was unable to go to college—her brother needed the meager family income for medical school. So my college education was an absolute. However, she thought of it only as an important part of being well-rounded so I could attract the right kind of husband!

I was a pretty feisty kid and used to argue with my mom because I wanted to be independent and be allowed on the same path as my older brother. My dad was always the one who remained calm and reasonable, encouraging me to be the best person I could be. Because I knew I was as smart as my brother, who was going to Yale, I worked hard and was accepted at Smith, one of the Seven Sister schools, equivalent to the Ivy League boys' schools. You might say we had some major rivalry going on, at least in my eyes.

During the holidays of my sophomore year of college, I had the best, most adult-feeling conversation with my dad I'd ever had. Then, shortly after I returned to school, I learned he had passed away while on a cruise. I lost my rudder and felt so alone. My mentor and counselor was gone.

I mentioned having lost much of my hair in my teens. This was devastating for my self-esteem. Funny how we dwell on the negatives and ignore all the signs that tell us we are really okay. I was very active and successful in school, and even became a cheerleader, and later learned at high school reunions that I was actually well liked. I never saw myself that way — the hair loss just made me feel so unattractive and unlovable. I bring up these memories because they set in motion how I was to feel about myself for years.

How do you feel about yourself? What self-doubts have held you back? Are you on the path to achieving your dreams or do you have a constant conversation in your head telling you that you can never get there?

When the women's and civil rights movements came along in the '60s and '70s I was married and living a life filled with all the things my mother had envisioned for me:

wifehood, motherhood.... I wanted so much to be a part of both those movements, but I didn't have the nerve to really do much about it other than in my mind. I called myself a "closet hippie" while I watched my younger sister act out the independence I dreamed of. I felt less and less freedom. My dreams and values stagnated as I watched the world go by. That limited sense of ME fueled me through my twenties and thirties.

Where Are You Now? Exercise

How about you? Before you do this exercise, think about these questions:

- Do you feel good about yourself and your accomplishments?
- If so, is where you are now where you still want to be?
- Have you found your purpose in life? Do you know why you were born in this time and what you are here to do?
- What is your attitude toward aging? If you are under forty, have you avoided thinking about getting older? If you are over forty, what thoughts run through your mind? What do you see when you look in the mirror, and how do you feel about it?

If you are over sixty-five, these questions are still vital—please don't discount them. In my seventies, I have many dreams and goals. You are never too old for them. Your dream might not be to climb Mount Kilimanjaro or run an eight-minute mile; maybe you just want to play golf every day or sit on the beach with a good book. Or you might want to write a book and change the world. All of these are dreams and goals. They count!

The First Step in Your Journey: As a first step, make two columns on a sheet of paper. On the left side, write down your dreams. Don't hold back. If you could choose the life you want most of all, what would it include? What places would you travel to? Who would you spend time with? What would you do with your time? Where would you live?

Then, on the right, list what is holding you back. This might be your own thoughts, your boss, other people, your age, your finances, your weight—whatever you *feel* is stopping you.

This list typically reveals how you feel about yourself. Here's an example:

My Dreams	What's Holding Me Back
To have my own successful business	No money to invest
To be 118 lbs., toned, and strong	I hate to exercise
	I'm lazy
	I don't think I have the discipline

In 1981 I was heading to a wedding, and not feeling very excited about it after having been through two divorces. I went to a nearby mall to pick up a card and bumped into a high school friend who'd married a close buddy of my first husband's. She showed me pictures of her two boys, same ages as mine, on a camping trip with their dad. My first husband didn't make his boys a priority in his life and would never have considered doing something like that. Tears rolled down my face thinking of what they had missed and how unhappy I had been. She turned to me with compassion and said, "We never understood why you married him. You had everything — good family, good looks, a great personality, intelligence."

"I never saw myself like that," I replied.

What had held me back? What was going on that I made those choices? When I started to understand more about my lack of self-esteem, my fear of society's disapproval, and the absence of my dad at an early age, it began to make more sense.

Because I had no real mentor, after I returned from Brazil and ended my second marriage I sought counseling to help me sort out why I felt unworthy and undeserving — why I felt like I wasn't enough. Today I might do it differently, but therapy helped me and I believe it can be very beneficial.

What are you thinking and feeling about yourself that may or may not be true, and how has that impacted your life? Ways to get at your core issues include building your own support group of trusted friends, writing in a journal, or creating a daily gratitude practice. Alternative therapies like hypnosis can also help you identify and heal what is limiting you. I list more of these in chapter 3.

As I learned more, I shifted how I looked at my life. This meant remembering that I am not my body but I am a soul/spirit in human form, and that my body is like my car and I am the driver. I love what Joel Osteen said: "Life doesn't happen to us. It happens for us." I started to see everything I'd gone through not as failure or success, but as the wonderful tapestry that makes up ME.

I address this more in other chapters, but with that in mind, I want to give you an additional exercise, one that saved me countless times from falling into the pit of sadness, anger, or depression. Here are a few questions to ask yourself. Take some time to answer:

- Do you have good relationships with partner and family? Could they be better?

- How is your health? Do you have lots of energy and vitality? Do you jump out of bed, ready to face the day?

- What stresses you the most?

- What depresses you most or makes you feel sad?

- What do you do for fun? Are these activities you have always loved and made time for, or have you abandoned those because of obligations and duties? What activities are you missing?

Now create those two columns again. On the left side list all the things, events, or people that anger or depress you. These might include coworkers, relatives, your physical health, politics, medications you resent having to take, your weight, or your financial situation. Now on the right side, list something for which you can be grateful in each situation on the left. Here is an example:

Things/People that Upset Me   Being Grateful

A nasty, sarcastic first husband   I learned to stand up for myself

When I knew I wanted to divorce my first husband, I went back to school and earned my certified public accountant (CPA) certification. Much later, when I returned from Brazil, I took a corporate job in accounting. After several years I felt bored, no longer liked that job, and started looking for a new one. When a job opened with the human resources and payroll company ADP to market their payroll software, I thought it was perfect. I had made it to the final four when they told me I that my lack of a marketing background disqualified me. I was so disappointed and depressed.

What ended up happening, however, is that I became interested in building my own business, which gave me the time, flexibility, and income I needed to live the way I wanted to. And I started to build that business while I still had the accounting job. I worked in the evenings, during my lunch hour, and on weekends. Keeping that boring job became one of the best things in my life. It didn't happen *to* me... it happened *for* me.

How about you? It's easy to rant and rave about people, situations, and experiences, but what happens when you switch to gratitude for what they have brought you in the long term? If you start to look at "bad" things with a different mindset, you are well on your road to freedom and balance.

What does all of this have to do with vibrant and joyful aging?

Have you ever noticed how stress ages us unless we know how to manage it? You know when people have been through a tough year, a period of grief, or a time of anxiety; they look older, grayer, and more tired.

When I was studying accounting, I had a part-time job at an accounting firm. Once I was sent to a woman's home to deliver papers. When she opened the door, it was as though a blast of dark, angry air spewed out at me! I was caught by surprise. Within minutes of handing her the papers, she was telling me about the awful husband she was divorcing and how everything in her life was horrible. She looked old and shriveled, though I know she couldn't have been more than forty.

The image of this woman has remained with me. And one of my biggest secrets for staying youthful is remembering that how I handle disappointment, grief, and anger shows up on my face and in my body. Changing my mindset and focusing constantly on what I've learned and the opportunities I've gained has shifted my life to one that is more beautiful and abundant and has given me a more grateful, positive outlook. This is much of the reason I look and feel younger than my age.

Now that you know where you are beginning on this journey, we're ready to get more specific. I am so excited to share with you the strategies and ideas that have been important to me in getting healthy and looking younger than my years. I invite you to join me in creating your own version of optimal well-being every day of your future life!

Take a look at the lists you created. How much of what limits you comes from what you have learned from family, friends, and your environment? Is it time to unlearn many of the ideas that have held you back and relearn some new ways?

CHAPTER 3
WHAT YOU THINK IS WHAT YOU GET

"It's My Life"

It's my life
And it's now or never
'Cause I ain't gonna live forever
I just want to live while I'm alive

— Bon Jovi

Every day,
think as you wake up,
today I am fortunate
to have woken up.

I am alive,
I have a precious human life.
I am not going to waste it.

I am going to use
all my energies to develop myself,
to expand my heart out to others,
to achieve enlightenment for
the benefit of all beings.

I am going to have
kind thoughts towards others.

I am not going to get angry,
Or think badly about others.

I am going to benefit others
as much as I can.

— *His Holiness the XIV Dalai Lama*

When I was twelve and in my third year of sleep-away camp, I was very competitive. I loved sports and played to win. When another camper on my team missed a ball or made a bad shot, I would get so angry. "They are so bad!" "How stupid was that shot?" "Why did I get stuck with them on my team?"

For participating and succeeding in different activities, campers earned yellow felt sun rays we glued onto a large dark-green background to build a sun. I *desperately* wanted that sun. The rays were handed out at one of the last camp events. I waited to get mine — positive that I had earned each one. After all, I was so good at sports! The only problem was that you could not complete your entire sun unless you earned the most important ray, the one for sportsmanship and cooperation.

I was so disappointed and embarrassed when my name wasn't called for this ray. But I quickly realized I didn't deserve it. I made a vow that I would come back and earn it the next year.

You know that phrase "Fake it till you make it"? Well, the next summer I did just that right from the first day of camp. "Nice try!" I called to other players. "You'll do better next time!" I said when someone missed a shot. "Can I help you with that?" I'd offer when we were putting away equipment.

As the summer wore on, though, I wasn't faking; I began to really mean it! When I messed up and someone encouraged me, it felt good to have that support behind me as well. I began to understand the importance of building relationships based on how others feel, not just on my own selfish feelings or desire to win. I also began to get out of my own ego when dealing with others, be more neutral and thoughtful, and eventually not take things so personally. On the last day I was so proud to collect my final ray and complete my sun.

That summer camp experience has stuck with me for a lifetime. Today I feel very good about my relationships and maintain an optimistic, encouraging attitude toward life and others. And I have also been taken advantage of and made some poor decisions along the way. As I have grown older and wiser, however, I see how I grew from these experiences. Instead of complaining bitterly and neglecting the lessons learned, I now look at people and things with a more discerning eye.

We humans are such a complicated bunch. (Maybe that's why this is almost the longest chapter in the book!) It's easy to look at people and events and be filled with anger, hurt, sadness, and disappointment. That's how our world is geared, isn't it? So many conversations are focused on gripes, resentments, and hurts. It takes a lot of intention to be compassionate, caring, and forgiving toward those who have made our lives hard. Life gets a bit more complex than summer camp!

Those old negative responses are based on our egos and our expectations that others should always be aware of our feelings and our wishes. Think about how many conversations include phrases like "Can you believe he did that?" and "Can you believe she said that?" We expect others to act a certain way—and when they don't, well, good luck to them! However, when our perspectives change, our attitudes change, and it is amazing how much happier we can be with ourselves and others.

Why do we develop bad attitudes in the first place?

You don't have to be a psychologist to see how easy it is when we are young to begin to not trust ourselves, to not feel good enough, and to have self-talk that spews out self-criticism and self-doubt. Some children constantly hear things like "That was so stupid!" "Don't you know any better?" "You're ugly and fat and dumb," or some other degrading or negative comment. Sometimes it's more subtle. Perhaps your parent sharply told you to be quiet when you were singing or playing joyfully... when you were feeling good and happy and just expressing yourself. It really doesn't take a whole lot to turn a person against themselves.

My mom was that critical voice. I can't count the number of times I told her something and she said, "That's the most ridiculous thing I have ever heard!" And though I was never heavy, she often cautioned, "Joanie, don't eat THAT! You've already been putting on extra weight." As a grown adult, after years of wearing a wig or hairpiece to cover my thin hair, I made a decision to no longer wear them. My mom would say over and over, "Why don't you get a wig? You look so good in one." Wow, did I look *that* bad without them?

While my subconscious totally absorbed these types of statements as truth, I consciously ignored them. Little did I realize that I became my very own critical voice, bringing down my own self-esteem for many, many years.

When I began my personal journey at age forty, I started to shelve those stories the little girl inside me had held on to. Now I have new, more rewarding and affirming perspectives and beliefs. Not that those old ones don't jump off the shelf on occasion, but that happens less and less frequently. (And now, by the way, I do wear wigs, but only when I feel like it and without their becoming part of my identity.) I lived long enough with that nagging self-doubt, fearing I would be found out, dreading the moment that the other shoe would drop. I know today that I am a strong, often opinionated woman who is empowered to fulfill my purpose here no matter what's going on around me.

Some are able to see their growth right in the moment, some aren't. It doesn't matter; start where you are! If you can't see it, ask your best friend to tell you how awesome you are!

There have been times in my life when it was challenging to give myself credit or feel good about what I had accomplished. In 1975 I was determined to get out of my emotionally abusive first marriage. Not only was I constantly ridiculed, but my husband also berated my older son with negative, sarcastic remarks. My parents didn't like visiting because of the nasty mental abuse he gave my son about almost anything my son did, good or bad. It was painful to witness, but I didn't have the courage to fight it.

Finally, when I knew I wanted to divorce, I had to find a job that could support me and my children, just in case there was any problem receiving child support. Because a neighbor taught accounting at the University of Maryland and I had always been decent in math, I decided to go back to school in accounting. I had no support at home so I only took one class at a time. My husband made snide comment after snide comment about my schooling, but I was determined. In my early thirties by now, I was glad to have fellow students to explain some of the more complicated concepts I'd forgotten over the years. As I was finishing my last class, I told my husband I wanted to separate. Finally I would be on my own. I finished my classes and later passed my CPA exam.

I tell you this because at the time I didn't give myself credit for the effort it took to run a household with two children, fight off a spouse who totally opposed what I was doing, and get all A's in my courses (well, except for statistics and IT—and I got Bs in those classes!)

Do you give yourself the credit you deserve?

I get that it's hard to feel accomplished and very easy to look only at the negatives and mistakes. A few years later I found myself in Brazil, where my boys and I had moved with my second husband. After all that drama in my first marriage, you'd think I'd choose my next husband more wisely. Nope. Not the case. The marriage was failing, and for two months I had been trying to leave, but the travel laws required a husband's permission. One day he'd say I could take everything with me; the next, nothing; the third day he wouldn't even talk about it. My boys were already back in the US at boarding schools and my husband was trying to convince me to let them live with their father instead of us. There was no way that was going to happen.

Finally he provided the official permission and got me a ticket. I took the dog, two boxes of household goods, and a very heavy carry-on with all my good silver and jewelry. I felt like a bag lady, but was so happy to leave.

I thought that was it—I had stood up for myself and made my break, after all. But that whole trip was to be a lesson in continuing to stand up for myself. First our armed driver, who had been with us the whole time I was in Brazil, pleaded with me to have sex with him on the way to the airport. Shaken, I calmly talked him out of it, said goodbye, and breathed a sigh of relief when he left.

Then, after a hair-raising engine fire (complete with passengers praying the rosary in Spanish and some hysterical screaming) and an emergency landing at the smallest airport ever, the hotel to which we'd been sent refused to take my dog. That wasn't going to happen! Again I stood my ground.

We were in that small Brazilian town for twenty-four hours before another plane came to take us on our journey. I had missed my flight to DC, which only flew once a week. The new plan was to wait two days in Lima, Peru, and then take another two flights to get home. Time to stand up again! I argued to get different flights after I was told I'd have to stay. Finally I made them put me back on the replacement plane, which was headed for California and closing its doors. Back in the US, I finally got on a flight from L.A. to D.C., still dragging along my dog, two boxes, and my heavy carry-on.

To top everything off, we landed in a snowstorm. I managed to hail a cab and endure a harrowing cab ride to my mother's. And yet I was still standing!

Within two weeks I had a job, a car, and a new place to live. As I look back, I am amazed that after such a shaky time in Brazil I got so much done so quickly and did what was needed for my kids and me. It was only possible because I was slowly beginning to recognize my own value.

It wasn't until five years later, however, that I truly got on the fast track to self-worth. Three years later I had major surgery and just could not get my energy back. I gained weight and felt miserable. My doctor told me that all of this was "natural" since I was over forty and had had surgery. What???

This provided me with another opportunity, this time to learn about building wellness through nutrition. I was not unfamiliar with this concept, as I had tried to help my older son conquer ADHD years before. Two years later I decided to turn my love of nutrition and wellness, rekindled after that surgery setback, into a business with the products that had changed my health. At that point I didn't know that personal growth and development counted for at least 50 percent of success in any business. I started to learn this very quickly. I got conscious about setting goals and affirming my ability to reach them.

One weekend a friend invited me to go to a spiritual retreat in Massachusetts. A fateful encounter with a couple at the retreat opened the door for me to meet two people who would become my spiritual teachers. I still work with the woman of that couple to this day, thirty-plus years later! (Her husband passed away several years ago.)

They taught what I call "practical spirituality." I learned to look at who I was being – spiritually – in my day-to-day life. I learned the principles I still follow every day. I discovered how powerful my thoughts and beliefs are. I started seeing my life as something I was creating every day and that I was responsible for every single result that showed up for me. I started working with my emotions. These concepts fit right into my new business in health and wellness, and truly transformed my life.

I have now been in business for more than thirty years, and each day I know that without all those experiences I would have had a very different outcome. I would not be a seventy-four-year-old with energy and optimism, inspiring others. By taking responsibility for my thoughts and actions—bye-bye "Blame Game"—life has more clarity and my attitude remains upbeat and positive. I know I am (and we all are) so much more than just this human form.

If you are hard on yourself—if you listen to that inner voice telling you that you are not worthy, not deserving, and not enough—please let this be your wake-up call. Those feelings are just feelings.

Changing your attitude is not a single one-and-done action. Here are all the tools I use on a regular basis to keep my perspective youthful and happy:

My Attitude Toolkit

Many have asked me how I keep my positive attitude. So I put together this toolkit to help you minimize "brain trash" and handle life's diverse events.

1. Document Your 100 Gratitudes

A major part of my growth was learning to be grateful. I really am thankful for all those missteps and poor decisions.

Without them I would not be who I am today. I am also grateful for the wonders of each day and the little things, as well as the big events and people in my life. Savoring each moment—whether it is kicking the soccer ball with my grandson or receiving an award on stage—creates more joy, gratefulness, and acceptance in my daily life.

Sit down with a pad and pen and begin writing down all of the things you are grateful for. Try to write one hundred of them: seeing the sun in the morning; the beautiful trees around you; a baby's smile. If you have been depressed and down on yourself, this is a great place to begin. Consider the people in your life and note what you are grateful for in those relationships. Even in the worst relationship you can be grateful that you recognize that it is not what you want or deserve. Be grateful for that recognition and that you can plan to move on or change it.

2. Continue to Write Your Daily Thank-Yous

To set your day each morning, write down at least five things for which you are grateful. Begin with: "I am grateful for ____," then add "because_____." At the end of each, write "Thank you, thank you, thank you." You will be amazed at how you feel after the first few days. This can also dramatically improve your challenging relationships and make your good ones even better.

3. Look in the Mirror

This one is not easy at first. Look in the mirror and say, "You are beautiful and I love you." I first did this "mirror process" at a workshop at which we were given mirrors and had to say this repeatedly. I bawled through the whole thing—I didn't feel beautiful then and didn't really know whether I loved myself or not.

Please do this! Daily. Because whether you feel too fat, too thin, too old, or too gray, you ARE beautiful. You deserve to love who you are right now and not withhold that love. I can't stress how important it is to do this every day in order to bring out the beautiful person you truly are.

4. What's Bugging You?

Make a list of the things and/or people that bother you, whether they are tiny pet peeves or major frustrations. How do you normally react when these things happen or you see these people? How does your body feel? Take time to observe yourself and see if you can then determine where that upset or feeling comes from. When you feel jealous or envious of someone, what is it in your conscious or subconscious that is bringing these things up for you? What do you want in life that you don't have? It is our subconsciouses that create our outcomes.

How you view other people and situations is often a direct indication of how you view yourself. For instance, I normally don't have road rage—even a minor form of it. When I'm late, however, you are likely to hear me ranting and raving out loud at the car in front of me. Is it the slow driver's fault? Should I take it out on them because I'm late? And, of course, when I'm late is when I hit all the red lights! Today I take responsibility for my actions and reactions and remind myself that I am the cause of what has just happened. Instead of unraveling, I tell myself, "Just suck it up, Joan, and accept that you're going to be a few minutes late."

5. What to Do When You're Dissed

What if someone says something disrespectful or is critical of something you have done? You probably feel hurt or angry, right? Where does that come from? Were your parents critical of things you did as a child? Did this bring up other old issues? When you have a strong reaction or feel triggered, try to remember the first time you felt this way. Observe the core issue so you can understand and deal with it directly.

I am not saying to ignore someone's disrespectful remarks. It might be appropriate to say something like "You know, that remark is really rude and disrespectful. If this is the way you choose to talk to me, I think this conversation is over." You could add, "I would be happy to talk to you when you are in a better mood or can speak appropriately." If you can be neutral, especially as you begin to recognize the core issue in yourself, you will be able to keep calm and not use up all your energy in anger. Stand your ground, too. You deserve to be respected, and following through helps you believe that. If the rude remark is undeserved, it is THEIR issue, so mentally or verbally give it back to them!

A few years ago my adult son yelled at me for something I did. I knew his perception of the situation was incorrect and I had done nothing wrong. Instead of taking his anger on, after hearing him out I told him it was his issue and I knew I had done nothing wrong. I said I was giving this anger back to him. He could be as upset as he wanted but I was not taking it on! He was very surprised but it did end the conversation.

6. Watch Whom You Hang Out With

How do you spend your time? Do you spend it with people who complain, who are critical, who only see that life doesn't work? Do you feel good when you're around them? Do they meet your needs and support your goals? What are their lives like? Are they successful, healthy, and generous? As author Jim Rohn writes, you are the average of the five people you spend the most time with. These are the people who reflect you the most and the ones you become most like. Choose those folks you truly want to be with, using your inner wisdom.

7. Practice Your Passion Plan

Make a list of what you are passionate about. What really gets you excited? How does that fit into your life? Are you doing some of those things now? If not, why not? Create a life plan that includes what you love. If you are in a job you hate, use it as a scaffold to get you where you want to be. Back when I had that accounting job I so disliked, I changed my attitude. I focused on knowing I was only there until I grew my own business, which I loved. This allowed me to go to work smiling, because it was really just a means to an end that would bring me joy.

How do you look at life?

A happy life is just a string of happy moments. But most people don't allow the happy moment, because they're so busy trying to get a happy life.
— *Abraham-Hicks*

Average people, and I'm talking about the 97% of society, let events shape their lives. It's exceptional people who are able to change their perception of challenging events and overcome them.
— *Jeffery Combs*

8. Dealing with Stress

Did you know that according to endocrinologist and researcher Hans Selye, persistent stress is part of the cause in 100 percent of all diseases (or "dis-eases")?

I spent a decade as a caregiver for my former husband. I felt the constant strain of making sure he had what he needed and keeping our life going. Before that I was always stressed out by marriage difficulties, divorces, and being a single working mom. Thank goodness by the time I was a caregiver I had learned about building health and connecting with my spiritual self. This totally saved me.

Meditation was how I calmed my mind, connected with my spirit, and helped myself relax. When I had too much brain chatter, I used a guided meditation on a CD.

I learned to make good food choices and take extra anti-stress supplements. Sugary foods cause inflammation and mood changes. I would often eat a sweet treat to help my mood, but any improvement I felt was short-lived. I now have my cravings under control thanks to making several changes. A high-protein diet made a difference. Certain supplements also helped tremendously: a complete B-Complex and a combination of nutrients with ashwagandha became my daily best friends. They are still there as I need them.

Leave limiting attitudes behind. While we all have to tend to our own limited thinking, I do believe our cultural mindset is changing. Women today can benefit from these shifting attitudes. While many women in my age group believed (and perhaps still do) that they needed a man to look up to, I see a change in my son's generation. With the Gen-Xers, at least among my son and his friends, I see husbands fully participating in their children's upbringing and family duties. It is beautiful to watch the respectful attitudes these couples hold.

9. Affirmations and Better Questions

Instead of affirming to yourself that you're a loser doomed to repeat the same old mistakes, or too old, or too heavy, try repeating affirmations like these:

I choose to live a positive life, making the perfect choices for my body, mind, and spirit.

I easily let go of the habits and attitudes that interfere with my goals and beliefs.

I am strong and capable and always learning new things.

I expect to feel physically good.

I am filled with youthful energy.

My mind is becoming sharper with age.

And if you tend to ask questions like "Why does this always happen to me?" and "Who would hire or love someone like me anyway?" give these questions a try:

What else is possible?

What am I not seeing here?

What can I add to my life now that will generate health and vitality in the future?

Life is about the choices we make... every day. We all have our own stories about our lives. Maybe it is time to review yours and see if the older, wiser you still needs or believes them.

I admit I have made some very poor choices in my life. I might easily have ended up looking and feeling like that poor woman I delivered the accounting papers to so many years ago. I am so grateful for the changes I made after age forty. But if I could do it again, I would have made them a lot earlier. I would have raised my children differently, spending more time working and playing with them and having a lot more fun. I certainly would choose different husbands!

You can dwell in the "shoulda-woulda-couldas" of your life, but if you want to age with a vibrant attitude, one that will help you look and feel younger, I suggest you keep in mind a very important fact: We are all doing the best we can at any given moment, and that includes you.

What does that mean? Stop blaming others. Don't be so hard on yourself! Pick up the pieces, see what needs to change, and take the action steps to change it. As Vince Lombardi used to say, "The future is now."

Your light is seen, your heart is known,
your soul is cherished by more people than
you might imagine…
You are far more wonderful than you think
you are. Rest with that. Breathe again.
You are doing fine. More than fine.
Better than fine… So relax.

— Neale Donald Walsch

CHAPTER 4

YOU REALLY *ARE* WHAT YOU EAT

"I Feel Good!"

*Wo! I feel good, I knew that I would, now
I feel good, I knew that I would*

— *James Brown*

My friend Lois suffers from rheumatoid arthritis (RA), an autoimmune disease. After years of experimenting, she's learned how to navigate the painful inflammatory flares by managing her diet. She knows that when she doesn't eat sugar and wheat products, she feels great. But even with that awareness, she can't seem to stay on this regimen very long before she starts craving breads and sweet rolls. After she indulges in the treats, she feels rotten for a week or two before getting back on track. Then in a few days she feels good again.

I can relate. When I stick to meals that consist of clean protein, fruits, and veggies, I feel energetic and lean. And when I indulge in certain dairy, wheat, and sugar products, it's not pleasant—I get stuffed, bloated, and gassy, and it shows up the next morning on the scale. Yuck! I don't like how I feel and I hate that my pants don't fit. So why do I do this to myself? Just like Lois—and maybe like you—I sometimes crave the very thing I know is bad for me. What is that all about?

Do you know people who constantly complain about the pains they have, how tired they are, how fat they feel, and how bad their sleep is? These are among the long list of complaints that people attribute to *aging*.

Really? What if—like Lois's RA and my weight gain—those complaints are not related to aging? What if they can be minimized simply by making better choices in foods and supplements?

They can. I admit that I have a long history of emotional eating and addiction to sugary foods, and that sometimes I just let myself give in to that candy bar or brownie craving and begin again the next day. However, I've got a big toolbox of nutritional tools that allow me to gain control over that hungry little girl inside who can't wait for her next hot fudge sundae. (One of my friends actually calls me "Fudgie" because of the time I finished off the delicious jar of hot fudge she brought me.) And these tools can help you, too.

By making very simple food and supplement choices, you can find immediate relief from those powerful cravings and the resulting symptoms. Working in this field for so many years, I've heard so many inspiring stories:

A few years ago a close friend and client was diagnosed with uterine cancer that had spread. She totally changed her diet and began using nutritional products, including a very powerful Shaklee antioxidant product called Vivix™. This allowed her to lower her cancer-related numbers substantially and stay strong through chemotherapy.

My friend Marti and her husband were part of a country-western dance class I taught with my husband. Every week she'd either miss class because she wasn't well, or she'd show up and cough through the class. One day she asked if I could help her feel more energetic. I arrived at our appointment with a bag of my basic supplement program, just in case she was ready for it. As I walked in the door she said, "I probably can't use anything you have because I'm allergic to four hundred and ninety-three out of five hundred things I have been tested for!"

We talked about her ongoing bronchitis, her high blood pressure, and how she was allergic to *all* the medicines her doctor had prescribed. I then opened a bottle of alfalfa, one of my favorite products for cleansing and helping with allergies and bronchial problems. She sniffed it and said, "I can take this!"

Marti was never allergic to anything I gave her, and within four months her blood pressure was normal and she had more energy than she'd had in fifteen years. I was so happy for her.

But it doesn't end there! Over the next two years she became stronger and healthier, which turned out to be more than just a blessing of good health. What she thought was bronchitis was actually congestive heart failure from a leaking aortic valve. When the valve finally began to completely give way, she had major heart surgery to replace it. She thanked me over and over for helping her get healthy enough to breeze through surgery and heal quickly.

The body has its own miraculous healing powers. Building healthy cells allows us to combat most anything thrown at us, and what we throw at ourselves! Please consider giving your body the opportunity to self-heal naturally by feeding it what it really needs.

Giving in to those cravings begs some bigger questions:

Why, in our land of plenty, do we make so many bad food choices?

Why is our culture overweight and under-healthy?

We have so much information and natural, healthy food available to us, yet changing eating habits and learning to make different food choices can be one of the most challenging things we set out to do. Why?

I have a few theories about this. It's very easy to find advice about what you *should* be eating—that is, more fresh fruits and veggies and lean protein. Right? You've read plenty about what you should and shouldn't eat. So I don't want to give you diet advice or sample menus. Instead I want to focus on something you may not have read much about. How **biology** and **food industrialization** could be leading you to eat the foods that make you gain weight, lack focus, and feel fatigued or grumpy.

The Main Culprits

I've been researching and experimenting with food and nutrition for thirty years, and here's what I've observed. The main culprits in our culture's growing obesity and failing health are *sweets and carbohydrate addiction, our industrialized food sources, yeast,* and *low thyroid function.* I told you this wouldn't be your typical diet advice!

1. Are You Addicted to Sweets and Carbs?

I have something to tell you that you might not believe. Craving macaroni and Oreos isn't our natural state. But thanks to all of the additives and extra sugars and fats in many of our foods, it's no wonder we have basically become addicted to candies, cookies, breads, and pastas. And honestly, food corporations love it! When we want more, we buy more. They have also figured out the right combination of sugar, salt, and fat to make our bodies want more and more, not caring about the damage it does to us, just wanting to increase their bottom lines. There is a world of yummy, fake, and overprocessed foods just waiting for us to come and chow down.

And those TV ads only fuel our hunger. Why wouldn't we want to go out and buy all of those goodies? We see happy, slender, youthful people smiling as they enjoy their delicious junk food. We want it, too.

There is only one problem — and it's a big one. While these foods might please our taste buds and improve our attitudes for a short moment, they destroy our bodies over time, contributing to all types of diseases, aches, pains, weight gain, and accelerated aging.

I know that bite of tortilla chip or swig of cola can taste really good, but is that what you really want?

I have a moderate addiction to carbs. I can devour an entire box of crackers or cookies within a day of bringing them home. So I don't bring them home, especially when I am under stress or using food as an excuse to not do something else. I know that once I start, it can be difficult to stop.

Can you easily eat an entire box of crackers in a sitting? If you have one piece of bread at a restaurant, do you want to gobble down the whole basket? In the book *The Carbohydrate Addict's Diet*, Drs. Rachel and Richard Heller explain how a carbohydrate addict's system works versus that of a normal person's:

> We have discovered [it is] the insulin imbalance that may be causing you to lose control; why your cravings, hunger, and weight gain are not your fault; and, best of all, what you can do about it.

The authors describe the actual metabolic differences between normal and addictive responses to food. Simply put, your system produces insulin when you eat to signal your body to take in food. The cells "open their doors" to allow the nutrients or "food energy" in to complete the process. Those with carbohydrate addiction produce too much insulin and the cells "lock their doors" or become "insulin-resistant" so the blood sugar or food energy can't enter easily. With too much insulin, also known as the "hunger hormone," in the bloodstream, you want to eat more. I am simplifying this, but you can see how it is different from the normal digestive process.

Are You a Carb Addict?

Take the complete quiz at www.carbohydrateaddicts.com/caquiz.html or in the book *The Carbohydrate Addict's Diet*.

Answer yes or no to the following few sample statements as if you were not on a diet or worrying about counting calories:

- I get tired or hungry in the mid-afternoon.
- It is harder to control my eating the rest of the day if I have a breakfast containing carbs.
- Once I start eating sweets, starches, or snack foods, it is difficult to stop eating.
- If I'm feeling down, a snack of cake, cookies, or starchy snacks makes me feel better.
- Now and then I am a "secret" eater.

If you answered yes to all of these, you are addicted to carbs. If you answered yes to three, chances are you have a carb addiction. If yes to none, you are doing well and have normal digestive patterns. The full questionnaire is very helpful, but only if you are honest.

The Hellers' program for cutting carb cravings might seem counterintuitive, but it works. The basic program: Through the day eat protein with only a small amount, if any, of low-glycemic carbs (see the chart in "Resources"). At dinner you can have your carbs with your protein.

I recently did a five-day reset program that is very similar to the Hellers' program, and the results were amazing. For the first time I didn't feel the need for sweets and breads and could walk right past them in the stores. I easily lost the last few pounds I'd been trying to lose and felt energized and satisfied.

You can find this program on my website and in "Resources."

2. Do You Know What's in Your Food?

Getting older can be joyful and relatively easy — or it can be filled with creaky bones, hot flashes, digestive problems, and sleepless nights. When you become more aware of what's really going on with the food you purchase, you can correct or even avoid some of those underlying physical causes as well as the symptoms that everyone claims are age-related.

A few years ago a massage therapist friend of mine suffered from hot flashes. She didn't want to take medication, so she began to research her options. Simply by changing her diet to all organic foods (and learning which of these to eat and not eat), she completely eliminated her hot flashes. There are also supplements designed for perimenopause and menopause that can help you if this is a problem for you. (See next page for the program recommended by OB-GYN Marcelle Pick.)

Eat Right to Prevent Hot Flashes and Balance Hormones

Protein is one of the raw materials for making and balancing hormones. Be sure to eat some with each meal and snack.

- Oatmeal with fresh ground flax and non-GMO soy milk
- Snacks: broccoli, cauliflower, or celery for dipping into a garlic tofu sauce; roasted non-GMO soy nuts; smoothie with deep-colored berries and non-GMO soy protein
- Essential fatty acids: fish oil, olive oil, nuts, and avocados. Omega-3s are especially important in balancing hormones. Be sure to use only highly purified fish oil, if that is your choice.
- Lots of veggies and fruits: whole so that you can get both fiber and phytochemicals, especially phytoestrogens for hormone balance (isoflavones, lignans, and coumestans). Cruciferous greens such as broccoli sprouts, watercress, collards, and kale, plus cabbage, Brussels sprouts, cauliflower, radishes, and their relatives work well.

Foods to avoid:

1. White sugar products
2. White flour processed foods like pastas and breads
3. Caffeinated drinks, chocolate, red wine, aged cheeses, and dishes that are deep-fried or overly spicy. These are typical hot-flash triggers for many women.

— Dr. Marcelle Pick, OB-GYN, www.womentowomen.com

Foods have changed over the last thirty years or so. We have seen the fastest growth in agricultural chemicals added to our planet's soil, including some 45,000 – 50,000 different pesticides with approximately 600 active ingredients. It is not unusual for fruits and vegetables to be sprayed ten to fifteen times before harvesting.[1]

I have kept an eye on this for years, and as a result I am very careful about where I buy my fruits and vegetables and where they come from. I know what is safe and what is not.

What about GMOs? The jury is still out as to whether foods that contain genetically modified organisms (GMOs) pose a danger, and there are no long-term studies showing the effects on humans of consuming GMOs. Many countries (currently not the US or Canada) restrict or ban the use of GMOs. But it's certainly worthwhile to research which GMOs might be safer than others. Here's my take on it: If a plant seed has been given components from fertilizers like Roundup®, I am absolutely not going to buy it. I am all for labeling that lets the consumer know what we are purchasing, but such labeling is not required currently.

So how do you avoid GMOs? Stay away from junk food. Buy food labeled "USDA Organic," as USDA Organic Standards prohibit the use of GMOs; many products labeled organic do not pass USDA standards, do not carry the "USDA Organic" logo, and *do* contain GMOs. (Most fruits and veggies are grown without GMOs

---

[1] http://www.living-foods.com/articles/poisoningfoods.html

but from genetically modified seed: corn, Hawaiian papaya, edamame (soybeans), zucchini, and yellow summer squash.[2]) Look for the third-party seal of approval "Non-GMO" label. Following are the Environmental Working Group's "Dirty Dozen" and "Clean 15" lists:

Dirty Dozen

- Peaches
- Apples
- Sweet Bell Peppers
- Celery
- Nectarines
- Strawberries
- Cherries
- Pears
- Grapes (Imported)
- Spinach
- Tomatoes
- Cucumbers

Clean 15

- Avocado
- Corn
- Pineapple
- Cabbage

---

[2] http://www.wholefoodsmarket.com/gmo-shopping-tips

- Sweet Peas
- Onions
- Asparagus
- Mangoes
- Papayas
- Kiwi
- Eggplant
- Honeydew
- Grapefruit
- Cantaloupe
- Cauliflower

It's not only produce and junk food that are risky. Consider the sources of your "real" foods, too. Beyond the Dirty Dozen, you also want to look into where your meat, chicken, and fish come from. Being aware gives you the knowledge to make good choices. You can decide what to purchase and consume, so why not have some awareness behind your decisions?

A few years ago I watched the documentary *Food, Inc.,* and it changed my life. Please check it out if you haven't— it's available at Netflix. I was so horrified to see what is happening in our meat industry that I now buy only grass-fed beef and organic chicken. I choose only wild fish, as I don't want to eat farmed fish that grew up in a chemical soup. But even making these very intentional choices, I never really know what has been crossbred or entered the lives of the animal products I choose. As far as I'm concerned, the fewer chemicals in my body, the better. My goal is to eat animal products as infrequently as possible.

I keep a copy of *Time Magazine's* 2011 health issue on my desk because the statistics boggled my mind. Get this: The nutrient value of our foods is 5 to 38 percent of what it was in 1950. Ninety percent of Americans fall short in getting essential nutrients in our diets. The increase in just ten years (1999–2009) in percentage of diagnoses of major diseases was 9.3 percent for heart disease, 19.6 percent for cancer, and a whopping 34.5 percent for diabetes. In that same time frame there has been a 2000 percent increase in the amount of fast food Americans purchase. Besides being low quality and having poor nutritional value, fast foods are full of bad fats, sugar, and salt, making us fatter and fatter and not keeping us healthy.[3]

"But this burger tastes so good," you might say. "And some nights I don't have time to cook dinner." These convenient choices might make life easier in the short term, but they are taking a long-term toll on your long-term health.

We do not have to be fat, diseased, and in pain. This is not how we are meant to age. I have seen too many people who have given up hope, who make no effort to turn their lives around, hanging on the belief that every ache and pain they experience is due to getting older. Yet they won't look at what they are putting into their bodies.

---

[3] *Time Magazine,* June 13, 2011, Vol. 177, No. 24. Various articles, "Health Special Report."

I want to feel great for years to come, and barring accidents, I finally know that I am doing what it takes to get there and stay there.

3. Do You Have a Yeast Problem?

One of the most widespread yet unrecognized problems is *Candida albicans*—an overgrowth of yeast in our systems that has been called "The Missing Diagnosis." An invaluable resource is Dr. William Crook's *The Yeast Connection*, which shows how excess yeast in our systems can be the underlying cause of so many issues for which we take medications. Dr. Erik Bakker, a naturopath from New Zealand who is a candida expert, provides some of the best information on yeast problems of any I have encountered. Find more information in "Resources."

Per Dr. Bakker, here are some of the many symptoms that can be caused by a yeast overgrowth:

- Fatigue, tiredness, or malaise
- Bloating, flatulence (gas), indigestion
- Food allergies
- Diarrhea or constipation
- Bad breath
- Smelly feet
- Carbohydrate and sweets craving
- Vaginitis, thrush
- Anxiety/depression

- Impaired memory, poor concentration, a "foggy" brain with feelings of unreality, and general weakness
- Toenail fungus
- Cystitis/urethritis (urinary tract infection — painful, burning, or "stinging" sensations when trying to urinate)
- Menstrual irregularities
- Hormonal imbalance
- Loss of sex drive
- Stiff, creaking, and painful joints
- Muscle pain
- Chronic sinus and allergy issues, multiple chemical sensitivities
- Mucus or catarrh, hay fever, sinusitis, persistent cough
- Heart arrhythmia
- Discolored nails, acne, and other skin eruptions (nail and skin issues are classic tell-tale symptoms of candida)
- Earaches, headaches, and dizziness
- Weakened immune system

The inability to lose weight can also be a symptom. One of my clients could not lose weight no matter what she did. When she began taking the probiotic I recommended, which helps crowd out excess yeast in the system, she finally began to lose weight.

If you think you might have candida, the complete candida questionnaire can be found at Dr. Bakker's site, www.yeastinfection.org/yeast-infection-evaluation-test. For a quick assessment, here are some of the most telling questions to consider:

- Have you been on antibiotics for an extended period of time?
- Have you used any prednisone or cortisone-type drugs, including inhalants and creams?
- Does exposure to chemicals, perfumes, fabrics, or tobacco smoke provoke symptoms?
- Are your symptoms worse on damp or rainy days?
- Do you crave or really enjoy sugar, chocolate, sodas, candy, ice cream, etc.?
- Do you crave or really enjoy breads, potatoes, fries, and chips?
- Do you crave or really enjoy alcohol?
- Are you fatigued and lethargic?
- Do you feel "spaced out"?
- Do you have asthma or allergies?

Tackling candida takes commitment and includes changes in food choices and adding supportive supplementation. You will need to see what works best for you.

There are many nutritional programs and supplements that help rebuild healthy microflora in your intestinal tract. These two products help kill yeast and are recommended by either Dr. Bakker or Dr. Axe: Canxida™ Remove and Shaklee Candex™, or a caprylic acid supplement. For nutritional support in building health, please contact me directly.

These are the basic steps to take:

- Minimize or eliminate alcohol and processed and refined foods.
- Eat more fresh fruits and vegetables; lean, grass-fed meat and poultry; and wild fish. If your problem is severe, limit your fruit to one per day.
- For some, going wheat- and dairy-free helps.

Most people with candida also have digestive issues such as leaky gut, so lightly steaming or baking vegetables is helpful and not as hard on the digestive tract as raw foods can be.

4. Is Your Thyroid Function Low?

When I hit puberty at thirteen, something was off. By the age of fifteen I had lost most of my hair and my period had stopped. My mom took me to a gynecologist who diagnosed me with low thyroid function, or hypothyroidism. I have lived with thin hair since then, and, especially as a teenager, have suffered with feeling unattractive.

The other difficulty I had was controlling my weight, and even though I never let it get out of control, I easily put on fifteen pounds and struggled to keep it off. While I started out with some thyroid medication at age fifteen, I stopped using it in college. And the physician I saw when I was in my early twenties didn't believe in thyroid problems.

For years my thyroid tests came out "low normal," but my symptoms persisted. I knew had a thyroid problem. I was so relieved when an endocrinologist tested me with a complete thyroid panel that consisted of three lab tests: TSH (thyroid stimulating hormone), T4, and T3—and my doctor finally agreed with me that my thyroid was underactive.

Fortunately, because I'd been falling asleep at work and gaining weight (now I know these were symptoms related to my thyroid condition), I'd already been motivated to begin my nutritional journey and had experienced an increase in energy and weight loss. (I had no support for any of this from my physician, by the way.)

Since taking nutritional supplements for many years now, I've had only a few minimal symptoms, even without corrective medication. If you experience some of the typical symptoms of low thyroid function or hypothyroidism, you might want to ask for a complete thyroid panel.

Symptoms of Hypothyroidism

- Fatigue – beyond normal tiredness
- Weight changes – slows down metabolism
- Constipation and inability to digest well
- Menstrual abnormalities – missed periods, lighter than normal
- Muscle and joint pain – muscle weakness, tremors in your hands, pain, swelling, and stiffness

- Depression – mild to severe, panic attacks, mental sluggishness, inability to concentrate
- Carpal tunnel syndrome

Thyroid concerns can also interfere with heart health and even mental function. As someone with a thyroid condition, I know it can cause constipation, higher low-density lipoprotein (LDL), and for some, anxiety, insomnia, and even tremors.

On the recommendation of my nutrition teacher and my naturopath, I have also added extra iodine and a product that has several vitamins and minerals plus L-Tyrosine, an amino acid. While this has helped me, you should consult your health professional and ask for testing to see if you need it.

One of the deficiencies that often shows up with thyroid problems is iodine — and some consider it an epidemic in the US. One of iodine's roles is to maintain a healthy thyroid gland. Insufficient iodine is also linked to obesity, cognitive impairment, heart disease, psychiatric disorders, and various forms of cancer. Iodine is also thought to help ward off breast cancer and fibrocystic breast disease.[4]

It took me fifty years to get my thyroid working properly. I still get it monitored regularly. If you have tried everything else to lose weight, and feel constantly tired and sluggish,

[4] Nancy Piccone. "The Silent Epidemic of Iodine Deficiency." *Life Extension Magazine*, Oct. 2011.

it's worth a blood test (for a thyroid panel) to see if a thyroid hormone deficiency might be your challenge. Again, please get tested before you make any changes on your own.

Is your life filled with energy, vitality, and a sense of purpose?

If not, wouldn't it make sense to take a serious look at your food and supplement choices to help you build optimal health and create a plan to reach your goal? I notice that many people, yours truly included, don't make a decision to change their habits until they have had a major wake-up call.

When I began this journey, I felt desperate and didn't know what to do. My wake-up call was how horrible I felt at forty, how much weight I'd gained, and the fact that I was going to lose my job if I kept falling asleep at work! Being able to change all that sounds like a miracle — and it was. When I added just a few basic supplements, my life changed, without thyroid medication. Within two weeks I had more energy and was losing weight *without doing anything else differently*. It wasn't until after my seventieth birthday that I started taking the correct amount of natural thyroid medication, which finally balanced my thyroid. The supplementation kept me going all of those thirty years in between.

Today I feel fit and fabulous. I dance, do yoga, and make the best choices in what I eat to ensure I will stay this way. It took my feeling really awful to begin this journey, but it doesn't have to be this way for you. And maintaining this level of energy and staying healthy is not time-consuming. I continue to do my research about supplements and my food sources. I make sure I'm not consuming chemicals. Otherwise, living this way has become second nature.

Ask people who are healthy and vibrant what they are doing. I was at a dance recently and spoke with a couple who are seventy-eight and eighty. They look fantastic, and are still sharp and intelligent. Every day they exercise, make excellent choices in what they eat, and keep their brains engaged by performing at senior facilities. What a delightful life they are living.

I met another woman at that same event. Slender, muscular, and a regular dancer, she is in her early seventies like me. All three of them are excited about life and look forward to what they will do next. Me, too! I hate to think what our stories would be like if we didn't make proper nutritional choices and have great attitudes.

About Food Supplements

You can begin a better food and supplement program at any age, but the earlier you start, the better. Maybe your genetics gave you a fast metabolism, so weight is not an issue. Or you have genes that keep you from getting sick easily. If so, you are very fortunate. I have a little warning for you, however. Per Dr. Christiane Northrup, up to about age forty, genetics are king. After forty, your **lifestyle** is what counts in how your genes express themselves. The consequences of all your decisions, positive and negative, begin to show up, and by fifty you might begin to see some changes you thought would never happen: a big belly, extra weight, more fatigue, digestive issues, or more infections, just to name a few. Dr. Northrup speaks about this and more in her books and on her website. See the link in "Resources."

When I first started taking the supplements, my boss was very happy to see me awake at meetings. And I was thrilled that my metabolism shifted and I began to lose weight. I wasn't even exercising, but the supplements totally shifted everything in my body. And, again, no thyroid correction!

Supplements — the *quality* ones — really do work!!

Why do you need high-quality supplements?

I wrote earlier about the declining quality of our food. When you're not sure about the nutritional value of what you're eating, wouldn't it make sense to find a guaranteed supply of essential nutrients? Of course, *guaranteed* is the operative word here. You want to know that the products you're using are made from pure, raw materials, are researched and tested for the right combinations, and are actually breaking down and being absorbed by your body. That should be easy, right?

Well, it's not. Over the last several years tests have shown that some supplements are contaminated with lead, PCBs, and other toxic chemicals. Other tests reveal that some supplements contain anywhere from 0 to over 100 percent of the labeled ingredient(s). Depending on the ingredient, too much can be dangerous. With too little or none, you have just wasted your money. I believe this is why so many health professionals are skeptical about using supplements to build health.

Low-quality, not-guaranteed supplements might not be doing anything for you, *so which ones will actually give you what you need and perform the way you want them to? How much should you take? How should you choose your supplements?*

A medical professional from Texas, Dr. Bruce Miller, sent letters to more than 300 supplement companies asking about their peer-reviewed, published studies (the highest standard of research), their clinical testing, and their quality control protocols. (See "Resources" for the questions he asked.) Only Shaklee Corporation answered. (See "Resources" for details.) He learned that most supplements are made by the same few companies, with a few exceptions, but just have different labels. There is minimal scientific research backing them. Those that do research often use research from other scientific papers and don't do clinical trials with their own products.

In an interesting experiment, Dr. Miller also dropped hundreds of multivitamins into his fish tank (without fish present!) to see if they dissolved. What happened was he ended up with hundreds of undissolved pills, just sitting there. And that is what they could be doing in your digestive tract: traveling right through you — undissolved!

My goal is to make sure I keep a supply of guaranteed, high-quality essential nutrients on hand in a convenient form so I don't miss anything any day. Bottom line: If it is going into my body, I want to make sure it's pure, it's potent, and it performs! Otherwise, why bother?

My Original Supplement Program

I still use these supplements today because they have worked so well. In "Resources" I share my complete program to help you with your own decisions. These are the three products that changed everything for me:

- A high-quality **soy protein drink**. Your cells are 40 percent protein; it's a major building block of good health. Many people worry about soy, but I am perfectly comfortable with it if it's non-GMO, water-washed, room-temperature-processed, and organic. I use it mostly in smoothies. If you're not a carb addict, add fruit. I often toss in veggies like spinach and kale, and add half a banana to mask the taste. The smoothie is usually all I have for breakfast, although in winter I might add the powder to a bowl of oatmeal for something warm. I sometimes substitute a non-soy protein called *sacha inchi*, a Peruvian plant.

- A complete **multivitamin/mineral** combination. I use the version appropriate for my age. Quality nutrients that are pure and tested for absorption make all the difference.

- A Shaklee proprietary nine-herb combination called **Herb-Lax®** for cleansing.

Within two weeks of taking these three products, I regained my energy, stopped sleeping at work, and lost weight because my metabolism sped up. I felt so amazing, and was just thrilled. The friend I bought these from had told me I could return anything that didn't work. Hah! No need for that. I still use these same products thirty years later.

Several of my other foundational choices are listed in "Resources." I've added more supplements over time as I learned more and as I aged. My favorite starter program that has worked so well over the years is called the Basic 5 + 2. It includes five basic supplements along with one or two extra depending on what you need. Here are the additional supplements in my starter program:

Cleansing nutrients:

- **Alfalfa** works for me as a cleanser and also helps me with allergies and as a natural diuretic, and just generally helps me feel great.

Foundational nutrients:

- The same complete, whole-food multivitamin/mineral I mentioned above
- High-quality protein powder to build healthy cells. One of my favorites is **Shaklee's Life Plan** shake. It includes one-third of the daily essentials plus extra omega-3, a prebiotic, and probiotics that don't get killed by stomach acid.
- **Herb-Lax**, described above in my original program
- **Vitamin C** provides extra help for the immune system and minimizes stress.

- **B-Complex**, which helps with stress and nerves.
- **Calcium**. I use a calcium supplement that includes nutrients that help with calcium absorption, including vitamin D3, magnesium, zinc, copper, and manganese, to help keep my bones strong.

I have also added the following:

- **Omega-3**. This essential fat, abundant in certain fish, helps make the blood slicker, has been known to blunt inflammatory response, and is great for the heart. I am very careful in choosing this supplement, as so many fish are toxic and not all companies are careful in how they check and purify their fish oil.
- **Probiotics**. These key microflora, or good bacteria, are part of a working immune function and healthy digestion. They are killed by antibiotics, steroids, and stress. As mentioned above, they also play a role in preventing yeast buildup.
- **CoEnzyme Q-10**. This helps the heart, boosts energy, and more. My version also contains resveratrol, a high-potency antioxidant.

So where to begin?

Why not start with an assessment to see where you stand now? Visit my website, www.joanlubar.com, and take my online assessment for free. When you sign up there, you'll also receive a free booklet called "3 Must-Dos for Healthy Living" along with a complimentary fifteen-minute session with me to help you plan your healthy future. Another questionnaire, the **HealthPrint™**, gives you a personalized assessment complete with nutritional information and a complimentary fifteen-minute session with me as well. To access that, go to www.jlahealthstop.myshaklee.com and click on the HealthPrint icon at the bottom.

The Life of a Cell

Imagine this: Your body is made of *trillions* of cells. I often picture all of these little moving dots, swirling around inside me, and consider how these trillions of little-bitty things work together to create a functioning body and keep it operating optimally as I age.

I think of everything they are doing... Maintaining a strong heart that sends blood surging through my arteries to feed all of these cells, pushes all the old blood and its debris back through my body to get rid of what it doesn't need and be cleansed and replenished, and goes back and does it all again; eliminating all the cast-off cells and organisms; and keeping my brain clear so it can process thoughts and send messages to make my muscles work and lungs breathe.

That is only a fraction of what these trillions of cells are doing for you.

The remarkable thing is that only one group of elements keeps these trillions of cells working well. That group is **nutrients**: vitamins, minerals, essential fats, oxygen, protein, and water. Your cells are only as healthy as what you are (and are not) feeding them. You really ARE what you EAT!!

And that, my friends, is why I watch what I eat and how I supplement.

CHAPTER 5

YOUR BODY WAS MEANT TO MOVE!

"Rock around the Clock"

One, two, three o'clock, four o'clock rock
Five, six, seven o'clock, eight o'clock rock
Nine, ten, eleven o'clock, twelve o'clock rock
We're gonna rock around the clock tonight.

— *Bill Haley*

When I was five, my mom signed me up for dance class. I took lessons in what we called Modern Dance (anyone remember Martha Graham?) and tap. I can picture the short white satin skirt with the sequined royal-blue sash, and the white satin top with the sparkly trim. I remember holding my huge smile as we all danced across the stage.

The seed was planted, and I have been passionate about dance ever since. I continued Modern Dance into college, and along the way I also learned ballroom dancing for those special bar mitzvah and confirmation parties. And of course there was all that rock-and-roll. I danced as much as I could. But then I got busy with marriage and kids and work. Like so many of us, I put exercise away. I was just so tired at the end of the day.

Years later, after my children had grown and divorces had opened up some time in my schedule, I began to dance again—sometimes with a date, and often just with friends at a bar where there was music and a dance floor. Because I wasn't doing much else in the way of exercise except the occasional game of tennis, I felt flabby and without a lot of stamina.

Then came the night my neighbor convinced me to join her for some country-western dancing. I had never been a fan of country music, so I thought I would hate it. But I was hooked after the first number! The dancing was similar to the casual ballroom dancing I had done through my teens and early twenties, especially swing. And the music wasn't the boring old "twang," but more like rock-and-roll with a strong beat.

At a time when life was stressful, dancing became my outlet. I went into another world and forgot everything else. Three or four times a week I'd go after dinner to blow off steam. My body and my stamina got stronger and I even made a new set of friends. Through moving my body and having fun, life was good again!

I still love to dance, and have danced in several ballroom events this past year. Mind you, I don't like to exercise at a gym, or even at home. Maybe like you, I've wasted a great deal of money on gyms I never went to! Have you ever signed up all gung-ho in the beginning of the year, only to slowly fade away within a month or two?

In *Rock and Roll at Any Age* we're talking about staying and feeling as young as possible as long as possible, right? And some form of movement is absolutely essential to creating a healthy, mobile, and happy body! My goal is to help you *want* to move! To not think about it as something you *have* to do, but as something you *get* to do. Yes, you *get* to move your strong, healthy body. It's a privilege — so many people can't. I invite you to put on the song "I Like to Move It, Move It!" from the movie *Madagascar*. When I hear that song, I can't sit still!

Let's talk for a moment about why exercise is so necessary for your health, your weight, your mood, *and* your youthfulness. Exercise contributes to:

- Better balance
- Better posture
- Increased blood circulation
- Less risk of stroke and high blood pressure
- Improvement in most chronic disease symptoms
- Less illness
- Improved memory, lower risk of dementia
- Stronger, denser bones
- Less body fat
- Better weight control
- Stress relief
- Better sleep
- Lowered risk of type 2 diabetes

- Improved breathing

- Less depression

- Reduced PMS and menopause symptoms

- Reduced metabolic syndrome

- Greater creativity

- Better sex!

Did I miss anything?

As I look at the list, I see so many areas in which moving my body has helped me. Remember that I said I wasn't exercising when I began my journey? And how I was heavy and couldn't stay awake at work? Since making exercise a regular thing in my life, I can see a huge difference in my weight control, posture, bone density, and stress level. How about you? I don't care what your size or your age, it's time to get up and move!

Dr. Christiane Northrup has three amazing, easy exercises to do daily that will change your life. She also has so much more to say about aging. You can find a link to her video in "Resources."

If you already love exercise and get plenty of it in your day, feel free to skip to the next section. If not, let's find something that will work for you.

Do you like music? One of my favorite discoveries is a special yoga system called Brain & Body Yoga (more about yoga later). One of the instructors has us start each class by dancing and moving to fun music. She says that dancing to four songs a day is a great way to include enough exercise in your day. Can you move to four songs a day? Give it a try.

Do you enjoy nature? Is your neighborhood beautiful or is there a park or trail nearby where you can feast on the beauty we have been given? Do you have a friend who might join you? Walking with someone you enjoy makes the time go by faster and is so much fun. Or maybe walking for you is a time to contemplate, relax, and feel peaceful in nature's healing power.

I have friends who started out with casual walking, then moved on to power walking, and eventually began to jog. One has even gone on to run marathons, something that was never on her bucket list. You might be surprised at how a walk around your block develops.

Are group classes your thing? If you are somewhat disorganized, like me, you might benefit from going to a group class. I love these because there is a set time to fit into my schedule and show up. So while I don't like going to a gym, I love classes like Jazzercise™, zumba, and yoga. Obviously the first two, and others like them, move faster and are more like vigorous dancing. Pilates, yoga, tai chi, and other slower modalities with lots of stretching build your strength and stamina. You can find group spin classes, group swim classes, and group weightlifting classes. Weight training and resistance work build bone density, which is so important, especially for women. If you're procrastinating about getting started, try a few classes and see what feels like a fit for you. I promise, even if you don't like the idea of exercising, there's something out there that you can do.

I have a regular dance and yoga practice that I love, but finally "succumbed" to a special strength-building program because I knew I was missing that component. Even though it only takes three minutes, I was still procrastinating about it. So I set up an accountability agreement with my granddaughter, and I text her to tell her that I have done my exercises. I include this as part of my morning ritual every day. (By the way, accountability like this is fantastic for those of us who tend to slack off.) I challenged her to do it with me, and some days she even does.

The Sassy Sage 3-Minute Strength-Building Program

All you need is a timer and a calendar. Mark off on your calendar each day that you have done your three minutes.

1 minute: **Push-ups**, either against the wall, on your knees, or full-blown.

1 minute: **Squats**

1 minute: **Sit-ups or Crunches**

That's it! You're done. Do what you can every day, and track it. I promise you will notice your improved strength. And, remember, it is JUST three minutes!

If you are self-disciplined (I am still working on that myself), you can exercise at home, choosing from an amazing variety of videos or online programs that keep your circulation moving and your body strong. But if you are self-disciplined, you are probably already working out regularly.

Again, your goal is not to finish a marathon — it's simply to find what works for you and "Just do it!" Even a little movement makes a huge difference. If you need someone to join you — support and accountability can often make the impossible become possible — ask your friends if they're interested in creating bodies that can last years longer, with flexibility, strength, and youthfulness. If you don't know anyone, check out some of the community centers or groups you could join to meet people with like interests. You will find the right person.

My body is my vehicle in this life, and I want to still be ballroom dancing in my nineties and beyond! And why not? I recently saw a YouTube video of a woman celebrating her one-hundredth birthday by getting out on the dance floor and doing the West Coast Swing. You go, Girl!

Stretching Out Your Youth

As important as it is to stretch at any age to prevent stiffening, as we age recovery takes longer and can be a bit more difficult. The nutritional support I take for recovery helps, but I can quickly tell if I've missed too many days working out. It takes me longer to get back into my groove and feel comfortable again. Stretching before and after workouts helps prevent stiff or sore muscles and keeps me feeling flexible. As mentioned above, Dr. Christiane Northrup recommends her own three easy exercises that help tremendously!

I've had a lower back problem since I was twenty-one. It is a structural problem—a vertebra slid forward in my lower back—and for decades I've had pain ranging from mild discomfort to sharp sciatica pain down my leg. I discovered a set of stretching exercises that, when I do them, really make all the difference.

What shocked me, however, was that once I consistently practiced my Brain & Body Yoga and regular ballroom dancing, I had relief that not only lasted, but also changed my posture and allowed me to actually stand taller. I'm also able to do things like vacuuming that used to hurt me. (Hmmm, not sure I want to admit to that… it's so nice when someone else cleans my house!)

Yoga provides a fantastic amount of stretching. Tai chi is another great way to stay healthy, flexible, and balanced as you age. I'm sure you've seen pictures of large groups of people of all ages doing tai chi in parks in China.

I encourage you to try one of these forms of exercise. They have truly been life-changing for me, helping relieve back and sciatica pain and strengthen my core. Exercise provides relief for those with chronic diseases and helps people recover mobility after accidents that have impaired their ability to move. I want to introduce you to two courageous women who faced disease and injury and found relief and recovery through focused exercise:

Meet Colette

I met Colette at one of my first country-western dancing experiences. No one had more energy, danced harder, or had more fun than she did. We became friends and I learned that she had rheumatoid arthritis. I was surprised when she told me that not too long before, her hands were knotted and she had trouble moving without pain. Determined to beat this debilitating disease without drugs, she went to the library and read all she could. Besides changing her diet and using supplements, she embarked on a serious exercise program that eventually turned into lots of dancing. When I met her, her hands looked totally normal — without a single knot. I would never have guessed she'd once been in so much pain and discomfort. While she still experienced occasional minor pain and her RA still showed up on tests, those painful symptoms were gone.

She always said, "If I can do this, anyone can!"

Meet Helen

Helen and her husband had ballroom danced for years. It was her true passion in life. When she was in her seventies she tripped and hit her head on a table. The hospital found some bleeding in the brain and operated on her twice. During the second operation she had a stroke. Her doctor told her she would never walk again.

But when you have a passion for something, it drives you. Helen was determined to get back to dancing again. She told the physical therapists in her rehabilitation center that they were not to coddle her, but work her until she could move again. There were days when she couldn't stand, but she forced herself to do it. Her doctor was amazed. When she got home, she set up a gym in her basement and worked out every day—much more than I could ever imagine doing! I met Helen when she was in her early eighties—and dancing again! She had only one residual symptom, a slight drag in one leg. She called me for nutritional help because she wanted to get rid of the last symptom and have more energy. She got better and better and I was able to watch her dance with her husband again.

Do you have high blood pressure or a family history of stroke? Exercise is so crucial for you. I know two people who, by running and doing Jazzercise, have lowered their blood pressure without drugs, which in turn has reduced their risk of stroke. Give yourself the opportunity to lower all of your health risks naturally before you choose the pharmaceutical approach. Our bodies are miraculous and do a great job of self-healing—but only if they are allowed to move as they're meant to.

What if you have some physical impairment—a physical disability, a weight issue, or an autoimmune disease that has kept you sedentary? Believe it or not, movement, along with changes in diet, supplementation, and attitude, can totally change your life.

Start slowly! What can you do now? Are you in a wheelchair? There are chair exercise classes. I used to teach them, in fact. Are you overweight and out of breath? Walk around your home, starting with just one or two minutes. Time yourself. Each day add a little more to your routine. You will be amazed! From walking to the corner, to around the block, to eventually power walking—what can you do to begin your journey?

Exercise is a stress-buster. Many people run to release their stress. I dance. I cannot feel or think about anything else but the joy of moving to music. At my worst times, dancing lifted me out of the anxieties of my life. When you move you build up endorphins, those amazing mood-boosting hormones. Movement can help you tackle major emotional issues.

I cannot motivate you; that is your responsibility. I only hope to inspire you. What will it take? Do you have to be in enough pain? Is there an event you want to go to and be able to enjoy? What do you want or need so badly that you are willing to make a commitment to yourself?

Now, how can you keep that commitment? If you need support, get it! How wonderful it will be to grow older and enjoy your life to the fullest! As you can see, moving can change your life. There are so many ways we can build health and maintain our youthfulness, and movement is one major component. I encourage you to get honest with yourself and set up a plan that works for you and your future self! If you need help and support, you can contact me or find a friend or personal trainer to work with. Then it's up to you... Just do it!

CHAPTER 6

HOW YOUR ENVIRONMENT AFFECTS YOUR HEALTH

"Earth Song"

What about sunrise
What about rain
What about all the things
That you said we were to gain...
Did you ever stop to notice
The crying earth, the weeping shores.

— Michael Jackson

Years ago I flew into Los Angeles for the first time and saw the brown coating sitting on the horizon—the nasty smog I had heard about but never seen in person. I couldn't imagine the people in that city knowingly breathing that air. And here we are thirty-six years later... with the same awful environmental problems and many that are even worse.

The thing is, sometimes we don't see it as clearly as I did that day in L.A. Environmental toxins are invisible and all around us. Even in our homes.

A couple I know was out to lunch with their three-year-old son when he began to cough. When they got home the cough continued, and his heart was racing. They finally took him to the emergency room to find out he had asthma. There was no history of asthma in the family.

Another friend's first baby was just a few months old when he developed a respiratory illness. For most of the next year he was in and out of the doctor's office with recurring symptoms. In an attempt to help him, my friend had been spraying his room and his crib with a popular disinfectant.

When both families discovered non-toxic, safe household products — for general cleaning, laundry, and dish care — the results were impressive. The three-year-old has not had a recurrence of asthma nor needed the medication for more than ten years now, and the baby's respiratory illness ended and never returned.

Amazing, isn't it? But not when you consider that more than 80,000 chemicals have been added to our environment over the last thirty years. Only about 4,000 of those have been tested for toxicity.[5]

We can't control what's in the atmosphere, but we can control what we use in our households. My friends' examples remind us that we need to be aware of what chemicals we are using that could be creating major health problems. And it's not just respiratory illnesses in question. Exposure to chemicals at home, outdoors, or at work may

---

[5] http://www.ewg.org/skindeep/2011/04/12/why-this-matters/

increase your risk for cancer and other debilitating diseases. Certain chemicals, including benzene, beryllium, asbestos, vinyl chloride, and arsenic, are known human carcinogens, meaning they have been found to cause cancer in humans.

Cancer risk depends on how much, how long, how often, and when you are exposed to these chemicals. *When* you are exposed is important because a small exposure in the womb, for example, can be more serious than the same exposure as an adult. The genes that you inherit from your parents also play a role, as well as how strong your immune system is.

In 2008 the costs associated with childhood diseases linked to toxic exposures in the US was estimated at nearly $77 billion. To understand just how severe chemical exposures have become, consider this: Each year a total of 9.5 *trillion* pounds of chemicals are manufactured in or imported into the US, which translates to 30,000 pounds per American.[6] Yikes!

Do you remember Dupont's old tagline: "Better Living Through Chemistry"? Back then I didn't bat an eye when I heard those words, but today I would challenge them! This is not better living. Instead of putting *more* chemicals into our lives and bodies, we should be living in harmony with the planet and making choices that keep our Earth healthy so we can breathe easier, stay healthier, and live longer and free from disease.

---

[6] http://articles.mercola.com/sites/articles/
archive/2013/11/13/worst-endocrine-disruptors.aspx

When Your House "Smells Clean"

People tell me they love to "smell the clean" in their homes. To me it's a bad smell. It means the home is probably filled with toxic cleaning products, not cleanliness. Many of those "good smells" are evidence of the toxins you have just spread around your home. Think about it: Why do you have to wear a mask or gloves or get out of the room as soon as you spray some nasty cleaner in the room? And why would you ever go back in that room and allow your kids and pets in there? There are cleaners that perform just as well and won't make you sick. And believe me, you grow to love a clean smell that is fresh and non-chemical.

Here are some examples of the toxins found in many common cleaning products and some of the physical symptoms they are known to cause:

- **Chlorine bleach**: eye irritation; respiratory symptoms, including asthma

- **Ammonia**: eye irritation, headaches, lung irritation

- **Petroleum distillates** (metal polishes): temporary eye clouding; nervous system, skin, kidney, and eye damage

- **Phenol and cresol** (disinfectants): corrosive, possible diarrhea, dizziness, kidney and liver damage

- **Hydrochloric acid** (toilet bowl cleaners): burns the skin, possible vomiting and diarrhea, blindness

- **Formaldehyde** (preservative in many products): suspected carcinogen; irritant for lungs, eyes, throat, and skin

- **Nitrobenzene** (furniture polish): shallow breathing, vomiting, cancer, birth defects[7]

You can check for other harmful ingredients that might be in your cleaning products at http://householdproducts. nlm.nih.gov/.

There's also a toxic load of fungicides, pesticides, and herbicides that ends up in our food, as well as many overprocessed foods that have little or no nutritional value but fill us up with calories. When we eat that food that's so readily available in schools, hospitals, assisted living centers, and grocery stores, we're not only overfed and undernourished — we're also toxic!

I want to repeat the most important message of this book: **We are responsible for our choices.** We owe it to ourselves, our children, and future generations to care for our environment in whatever ways we can as individuals. If each one of us does our part and cleans up our side of the

---

[7] The list was compiled from the following US government sites that all agree: National Cancer Institute (www.cancer.gov); American Cancer Society (www.cancer.org); "Cancer Facts & Figures 2009," American Cancer Society, 2009; CDC's Division of Cancer Prevention and Control (www.cdc.gov/cancer); US Mortality Data 2006, National Center for Health Statistics; U.S. Centers for Disease Control and Prevention, 2009.

street, imagine how many illnesses we can prevent! Imagine how much better we might feel, and how those aches, pains, and symptoms we attribute to getting older might either be minimized or disappear!

What You Can Do

So what are some of the things in terms of your environment that you can do to improve your life and your health and stay and feel younger longer? Here are some ideas:

1. If you smoke, stop!

I mentioned earlier that my dad died when I was in college. When he was just fifty he was warned to stop smoking or he would die—this was after a heart attack and a diagnosis of angina ten years before. He didn't believe the doctors and kept smoking his three packs a day. One day, several months later, he overexerted himself on a cruise and keeled over and died. This was devastating to our whole family, and I still miss him terribly. It was so unnecessary.

We know so much more about the dangers of smoking now, but people still puff away. More and more young people are smoking again. They inhale toxic, cancer-causing ingredients willingly, and once they get hooked the addiction is incredibly hard to break. If this is you, please get help and do whatever it takes to quit. You are worth more than your addiction.

By the way, did you know that smoking makes your skin look grayer and your wrinkles more pronounced? If you want to look as young as possible as long as possible (I know I do), stop smoking!

2. Be aware of all the products you're using in your home and office.

When you spray cleaning products, they usually mist back onto you. About 60 percent of what touches your skin is absorbed into your bloodstream. Is that something you want? Those sprays are also falling to the floor, and if you have little ones around, they are crawling around in those chemicals.

What are you using in your laundry? Many detergents and whiteners leave residue in your clothes, sheets, and pillowcases. As you rub against your pillowcases and sheets, that is also entering your body. Could this be part of the reason for the double-digit increase in asthma and allergies? We are breathing those chemicals all night.

We live in homes and work in buildings that are well sealed to keep out the cold and the heat and keep us comfortable. What this also does, however, is seal in whatever toxic chemicals are in your home or workplace. New carpets and furniture glues "outgas" into the air around us the chemicals used in producing them. I know people who have developed coughs and even asthma and allergies from breathing these. Several years ago the Environmental Protection Agency (EPA) had to move out of their new building because the toxic outgassing from their new carpet was making everyone sick. Even the EPA needs protection!

You can look for and request sustainable building materials, furniture, and carpeting that have not been treated with harmful chemicals. The demand is beginning to increase, and when more and more consumers demand these products, producers will supply them.

I use some outstanding economical and non-toxic home-care products that typically outperform the toxic ones (see "Resources"). Because you use them a little differently than the products you might be used to, you'll want to learn how they are the most effective. When you clean with them, you won't have to wear gloves or leave the room to protect yourself from caustic chemicals! You'll breathe better, get healthier, and feel happier! And you'll spend less money. These products last a lot longer, so are more economical.

Years ago a good friend told me how her chest always seemed to hurt when she was cleaning. When her physician checked her over, he found nothing. After switching to some of these non-toxic cleaners I recommended and getting rid of her old products, the pain went away. Was that just a coincidence? Well, a year later she was cleaning a cabinet and found one of the old furniture polishes she'd missed when she gave away all her old cleaners. She thought she'd just try it, and as soon as she began to use it the discomfort in her lungs began again.

The products you use in your home make a huge difference... in your life and in the planet's life. Our environment deserves better choices as well. Just imagine what is happening to our waterways and soils as we dump, flush, and rinse away the toxic residues from all our products. If we all changed to non-toxic products, one person, one family at a time, can you see what a difference that could make?

3. Know what you're putting on your skin.

Skin-care products, makeup, hand soaps, antibacterial gels... all of these are absorbed into your bloodstream. In fact, the reason doctors use patches to send medicine into your system is because they deliver the medicine very effectively. Our lotions and personal care products are absorbed into our skin as quickly as the medicine from those patches. Just like your cleaning products, you might like the smell of your shampoo and lotion, but it's worth it to your long-term health to investigate the safe and unsafe ingredients in your products. Please evaluate what you are using.

For years I've been loyal to a line of antiaging skin products that work incredibly well and don't send potential cancer-causing and other-disease-causing chemicals into my bloodstream. I list this line, in addition to a few other companies whose products I like and recommend, in "Resources."

4. Ditch the antibacterial soaps.

Unless you work in healthcare or where you can't get to soap and water, I encourage you to stop using antibacterial products. Here's why: You have a special coating on your skin called the *acid mantle*. It helps naturally protect you from bacteria sneaking in. Most soaps and body cleansers, however, are alkaline, and remove the acid mantle, making you vulnerable to absorbing whatever your skin comes in contact with. When you use pH-balanced products on your skin, you keep this safety net intact. To test this, pick up some pH paper at the drugstore and dab some products on it. It will tell you just how close your products are to being pH balanced.

One of the dangerous ingredients in antibacterial products is triclosan, a product added to prevent bacterial infections that once was only used by hospitals. According to LiveScience, many scientists now believe that not only is triclosan unnecessary for most household cleaning tasks, but it might contribute to the rise of drug-resistant bacteria. There are studies showing it can damage muscles and organs along with disrupting hormones. Outside of our bodies, triclosan reacts with chlorine in tap water, creating chloroform, which can eventually seep into our waterways. This is not a chemical you want to add to your toxic load. Besides, studies are showing that vigorous hand-washing with soap does a better job of getting rid of bacteria.[8]

I have just touched the surface of this global issue. What we each can do about it is simple, and urgent: We need to be aware of our environmental hazards and make better choices. From the youngest infants to the oldest senior citizens (who often haven't made the best or healthiest decisions), limiting

[8] http://www.livescience.com/32573-is-it-better-to-wash-with-antibacterial-soap.html

exposure to toxic chemicals can make the difference between a longer, healthier life and premature death. Reducing your use of toxic chemicals is a no-brainer, and acting locally — very locally, inside your own home — you can think globally (and feel a whole lot better).

I have made some major changes in my life — in how I eat, how I exercise, how I talk to myself, and how I spend my time. And I have to say that the changes I made in my home environment were much easier to make than almost anything else health-related. You clean your home, wash yourself, do dishes and laundry, and take care of your skin, all with products you buy as a consumer. Why not use natural products that can also protect you?

Why not eliminate those toxic products that are adding to our stressed and ill population by doing damage to our bodies?

Why not simply switch to safer, healthier, non-toxic products that are also often less costly than what you're currently using?

You will feel better, get sick less often, and look younger; plus you'll be a steward of our planet.

CHAPTER 7

GET A GOOD NIGHT'S SLEEP AND STAY YOUNGER

"Help Me Make It through the Night"

Come and lay down by my side
Till the early mornin' light
All I'm takin' is your time
Help me make it through the night

— Kris Kristofferson

I know how to ruin a perfect day! Well, I should say I used to know how. Back in the day I'd pack my schedule with many events, appointments, and workout time, go to bed too late the night before, and wake up at 3:00 a.m. thinking about everything I had to do and wondering why I couldn't go back to sleep! I would finally get some rest, but needless to say, it wasn't the quality rest I needed to prepare me for the day... especially a day as full as that!

I admit that even today I still have those moments, but after learning more about the importance of sleep I am much more careful about my pre-bed routine, how my room is set up, and what I am thinking.

Why is enough sleep so important? I have to share this list because it really was a wake-up call for me! (*Smile.*) Without enough sleep:

1. It is more difficult to handle stress.

When you're tired you have a lower threshold for irritability and impatience. I can remember coming home from work years ago feeling brittle. I would tell my children not to even talk to me for the next half hour. I needed to close my eyes and deep breathe in order to take on the evening after a long day.

2. Your memory is affected.

Enough with the "senior moment" comments. You can be more forgetful any time you haven't slept well, and it's physical! There are actually fewer connections between your nerve cells because you haven't had enough deep sleep to facilitate them.

3. Your concentration is off.

Can you relate to this one? When you're tired you can't focus, and easily get distracted. Whether at work or at home, this can definitely affect your productivity. And how about those disconnected conversations? Life is about relationships, and there you are with your mind wandering!

4. You are more likely to overestimate your performance.

What an interesting phenomenon. The day after I slept badly wouldn't be the day I would want to be reviewed by my boss! Overestimating how well you're doing can also set you up for automobile accidents and other kinds of accidents.

5. You're more prone to weight gain.

Not only do the hormones that tell you to eat stay at higher levels when you haven't had enough sleep, but you're also not manufacturing the hormones that help you stop eating, so you crave those sweet and salty foods.

Sleep is *not* a luxury. It is vital to get enough sleep each night. Obviously we can't always get in eight full hours — the ideal time for adults, but here are some of my time-tested ways for giving it your best try:

Just get to bed.

My goal is to get to bed by 10:00 p.m. so I can get up between 6:00 and 6:30 a.m. But I'm usually lucky if I'm asleep by midnight. I know the best plan is to have a set bedtime so my body can regulate itself. Of course that doesn't mean I always do what I know is best... I'm only human! But if my stated goal is to get to bed by 10:00, I'm likely to do so most of the time.

Check the cortisol.

A couple of years ago I had my cortisol levels checked. These are the hormones that increase during our "fight or flight" reactions, a.k.a. "stress hormones." Mine rose after 10:00 p.m., which explained why I always got a second wind late in the evening. So if I go to bed at 10:00, I prevent the second wind and have a much better night's sleep.

Avoid late-night snacks.

Avoid eating for a few hours before you go to bed. If you eat a late dinner or large snack in the evening, your body is still digesting food at bedtime, and that can disrupt you instead of helping you sleep. You might even have disturbing dreams. What you eat can affect you in different ways. A heavy, spicy meal such as curry or a greasy meal like a burger and fries can mess with your sleep. Try to finish your last meal about four hours before going to bed. A *light* snack in between is okay. Years ago I was on vacation in Greece and met a couple who wanted to take my partner and me out for a special dinner. We first went to their house, and they served us so much food there that I was already full when we left at 11:00 to go to dinner. Dinner was a heavy lamb dish, and I could barely get any down, but I forced myself just to be polite. I was so uncomfortably full the whole night that I couldn't sleep. I don't do that anymore!

Limit screentime before bed.

Did you know that the ionized radiation emitted from electronics can affect your sleep? Most of us have TVs in our bedrooms, and many people go to sleep with their TV on, which can only mean lower-quality sleep. Do you keep your phone charging beside your bed? By moving it just three feet away you are exposed to 75 times less radiation. I charge my phone in the bathroom, at least twenty-five feet away. I can still hear the alarm in the morning, and if I want to listen to some soothing music to help me go to sleep, I can hear that as well. I also put it on airplane mode to avoid the electronic waves. If I am staying at a hotel or somewhere where there is a TV in the bedroom, I unplug it.

And think about what you are watching before bed. Many of the more violent shows are on late at night, and the nightly news replays every crime in your town. Not the best material to which to expose your poor brain when it's trying to relax!

Remember the ambiance.

Your bedroom is supposed to be your restful haven, a place to wind down from the day, bring you peace, and help you sleep. If the TV is blaring with violent shows, and late-night callers can text or call you, how is that for preparing for a night of rest and repair? I love to have soothing ambiance in my room. The colors in my room are dark greens and eggplant, making me feel as though I am in a forest. I can just walk into my bedroom and feel the stress of the day pour out. What a wonderful feeling of calm and relaxation!

Don't work in your bedroom—or in your bed! If you work at home, do so in a different part of the house.

Pillow and mattress matter.

Choice of mattress is another important part of good sleep, as is the choice of pillow. One day I plan to get a bed that will raise up under my knees and also raise at the head level. Because of a longtime back problem, I never sleep on my back, but with an adjustable bed I think I could do that! Is your mattress decades old? Sagging? How supportive is it?

How about your pillows? If you have a bad back, and sleep on your side, you might benefit from a pillow between your knees. A chiropractor is a great resource for determining what is best for you in the mattress and pillow department. And they often sell special pillows with indentations that help keep your body in a better position during sleep.

Time your exercise.

Exercising every day, consistently, helps you sleep better because your body has used your energy effectively and moved all the blood around to keep you in better balance. When it is time for bed, your body is ready to rest. I try to do some form of exercise every day, although I don't always achieve that goal. At the minimum I do the three-minute routine I wrote about above. Besides helping you rest, exercise can also help lower your cholesterol. But avoid exercising right before bed, as that interrupts your body's transition to relaxation.

Relaxation

If I'm tight from the day, I do some yoga stretching and take some calcium and magnesium tablets to help relax my muscles. Both calcium and magnesium are great for getting a restful sleep. They can also prevent muscle cramps. When I have woken up with an excruciating cramp in my leg, I was usually low on magnesium and water. A quick trick to help relieve the cramp is actually counterintuitive: tighten the muscle and squeeze it with your hands. This provides instant relief. Then you can get up and walk to get the magnesium and water you need, and to mobilize the muscle back into shape.

A wonderful elderly client of mine had restless leg syndrome. She began taking my calcium-magnesium supplement and was able to totally stop her restless leg and get a full night's rest again. Her mood improved. I loved knowing she didn't have to use medications any more.

I also use a product called Stress Relief Complex by Shaklee Corporation. This unique product was the key to keeping me relaxed and able to sleep during the years I was the caregiver for my husband. Others use melatonin or valerian (sometimes with passion flower) to help them sleep. Every body is different, so it's important to experiment to find what works best for you. My goal is to stay away from drugs and find natural ways to stay healthy so I don't have to worry about chemicals in my body or side effects.

If I'm feeling wide awake, or wake in the middle of the night, I either read or do a crossword puzzle. I don't let myself get frustrated with the crossword puzzle; I just set it aside if I get stuck. I might also have a cup of herbal tea, such as chamomile.

In bed, I do a relaxing yoga exercise in which I tap my feet together. I don't know why this helps, but my yoga instructor swears by it! I can do one hundred taps very quickly and it seems to calm my mind.

Last, I do deep breathing and meditate, often being grateful for the events of the day. If it has been a stressful day,

I use the time to let the events go and ask for help while I sleep in resolving any issues or questions. Or I count down from twenty-five, picturing each number and saying something like "I am so relaxed and so at peace" after each number. I am usually asleep before I get to one! If you aren't used to meditating and need extra help, find a guided meditation CD to help you. They do wonders! Having a routine that works for you is so beneficial. For most of us, knowing what's coming next, especially when moving into relaxation and sleep, is very calming. No surprises.

Sweet dreams!

CHAPTER 8

NAVIGATING THE INTERESTING AND INEVITABLE EVENTS OF AGING

"Whatcha Gonna Do?

Whatcha gonna do when she says goodbye
Whatcha gonna do when she is gone
Whatcha gonna do when she says goodbye
Whatcha gonna do when she is gone

And all at once you're ready to hang it up
'Cause things didn't turn out the way you planned
And all your friends they're calling you a fool
'Cause you don't know a good thing
When you got it in your hands

— Pablo Cruise

"My joints ache because I'm getting older."

"My brain is fuzzy."

"I just can't remember — I'm having a senior moment."

"Oh, I'm too old to do that!"

"It's hell to get old."

Do you hear these complaints a lot? Or do you say them yourself?

By now I hope you see that you can minimize or eliminate the effects of so many things that people assume are the result of aging. There are, however, some things that we must accept will change as we age, no matter what. With care, modifications, wise choices, and a good sense of humor we can certainly minimize the impacts of all of these.

When I was in my thirties and playing lots of tennis, I played singles with a seventy-something-year-old man who had once been a great athlete but now walked with a bandaged knee and couldn't run. He compensated by being a *master* at slicing the ball short; making me run forward, barely getting to the ball; then sending the ball back to the other side in the back court. He always knew my options and positioned himself where I had to hit the ball to. He was a fabulous example of how modifications, experience, and wisdom win the day, no matter what's going on!

Ruth Heindrich started running in her forties. She was later diagnosed with breast cancer that had moved to her lymph nodes. After extensive surgery she completely changed her diet, first to vegetarian, then to vegan, and finally to raw. She is still running, very healthy, and has logged more than a thousand races. Oh, by the way, she's in her eighties now and still going strong.

Have you seen that Facebook video of a white-haired eighty-something woman on the dance floor? It's one of my favorites. She volunteered to dance with a ballroom dancer who had just finished a sexy dance demonstration with a young woman at a street festival. She walked over with her cane and he carefully began to dance with her. Then suddenly she tossed her cane away, took off her jacket, and they began an amazing Latin dance, including drops and turns that were fantastic. The message: Don't be fooled by assumptions about aging. We are so much more capable than we are led to believe!

A seventy-year-old friend of mine went on an outdoor adventure with her daughter for a week. They climbed mountains, swam, did yoga, and barely stopped the very first day. That evening the owner called the trip leader to ask how the "old lady" was doing. "What old lady?" he said. "There's no old lady in this group!"

These stories all show that there is so much within your control... but what about what I call those inevitable aspects of aging?

1. Oh, My Aching Joints!

Welcome to joint and muscle pain and the inability to move with ease. Chances are you will have some deterioration in your joints as you age, especially if you haven't been consistent with exercise and have experienced some muscle and bone loss.

Even though I started exercising regularly at an older age, I have increased my bone density and muscle mass and kept my joints working well. Mind you, my lower back has a structural malformation. But between Jazzercise, Brain & Body Yoga, and ballroom dance, my posture has improved. After going through the short-term aches and pains as my muscles got back into shape, everything is now working great! I pulled a tendon in my knee recently and was able to heal it quickly. Some pain flares up now and then, but that can be true for anyone at any age. I am grateful I know what to do to treat it with no (or very occasionally a low dose of) drugs.

One huge thing I have realized, however, is that I lose muscle strength and flexibility more quickly, so it takes longer to get back "in motion" if I miss too many days of some sort of movement. That I attribute to aging. But simply by exercising more consistently I can minimize the problem. Also, I swear by supplements for recovery to stay pain-free and bounce back after exercise. I use an after-workout drink and a hydrating drink during workouts that includes magnesium, which helps with cramping. Many people are deficient in magnesium, and I know the extra magnesium has been very helpful for me!

A Shaklee product that is super effective for recovery, according to Olympic athletes (and me!), is a unique, potent combination of resveratrol, transresveratrol, and other antioxidants and polyphenols called **Vivix**™. Athletes find that it helps them heal more quickly from injuries. I suggested that one of my customers use it before and after surgery, with his doctor's permission, and despite his age (seventy-nine) he healed rapidly. He has used Shaklee products for over twenty-five years. Find out more about Vivix on my website or in "Resources."

Over the years I have experienced some joint pain at the bottom of my thumb. Turns out lots of people do. I began using a joint-health combination of glucosamine hydrochloride; boswellia, a natural pain reliever; and other specific nutrients, and the pain is totally gone now! That product is also listed in "Resources." And yes, it's a Shaklee product, too. I mention these because I have had continued success with them for over thirty years.

My eighty-two-year-old cousin and her eighty-seven-year-old husband told me that they are able to keep going strong on a daily basis. Every day they stretch and every other day they go to the gym and work out. Even when they are traveling they do leg movements in their airplane seats and get up every hour to walk up and down the aisle! What great ideas! I heard about this right before boarding a plane for a return trip across the country. When I had flown in two weeks before, I could barely move my knee without pain after being so immobile for five hours. But when I employed their strategies during the flight, I got right up when we arrived. Pain-free, I easily walked out of the plane and traveled home.

You can experience new pesky pains as you age, but you can overcome most of them without drugs when you take good care of your body. Just keep moving and don't forget to repair!

2. When the Law of Gravity Appears on Your Face

I learned how to stand on my head years ago, and perhaps had I continued to do that every day, I might have fewer lines on my face. But since I didn't, I had to find another way to minimize those wrinkles. By the way, I like to think of those lines as the result of aging with joy, laughter, and experience bubbling over in the way I look!

Unless you want to be stretched and tightened, looking frozen in time without the magnificence of personality showing through (a.k.a. facelift), just enjoy those lines and use safe, natural products to keep your skin as young and glowing as possible for as long as possible. My friend who lives in Alabama swears that the humidity there does wonders for her skin. To replicate that climate, try a steam bath once a week, even if it's just holding your face over some simmering water with healing herbs in it. I use a clay masque and a skin polisher, which tightens and smooths my skin and removes dead skin cells, plus a nutrition-based line of skin-care products that helps rebuild and feed my skin from the surface inward. As I've said, most people are surprised that I am in my seventies, not years younger. Find my skin-care regimen in the "Resources" section.

Many years ago I visited a friend in the hospital. Her roommate's face was so bruised and swollen, it resembled a black-and-blue basketball. Her head was swathed in a big bandage dotted with dried blood. It was an awful sight! When I asked her husband, "Was your wife in an accident?" he laughed! "No," he said, "She just had a facelift." Any thought I ever had of doing that ended in that moment. I'll go for the natural way, thank you!

I'm going to say this again: **If you smoke, stop!!** Besides all of the internal damage and potential for devastating cancers, COPD, and heart disease, it makes your skin look gray and speeds up those lines and wrinkles.

Feed your skin from the inside. There are nutrients that help create smooth and bright skin cells, helping you glow even with an older face. See the next page for suggested nutrients, along with why I suggest adding them to your daily regimen as you age. Look for more suggestions on my website, www.joanlubar.com.

Attitude is another way to minimize the wrinkled look of aging. It takes only thirteen muscles to smile, but more than one hundred to frown. Keep up that positive, forward-looking feeling, remembering that each moment can be a great one — and it will show on your face. Leave the past in the past. People who keep on movin' on just have a glow about them.

With some conscious care for your skin and your mindset, you can look fabulous, no matter what your age.

The Sassy Sage's Favorite Nutrients for the Skin:

- **Adequate protein**, preferably high-quality, vegetable-based, because your skin cells are primarily protein.

- **Vitamin C**, the foundation of collagen, is the "glue" to hold your skin cells together; plus it helps with stress, which affects your aging looks.

- **Vitamin E**, with selenium, protects cell membranes, tones muscles, and improves elasticity. Be sure it is natural and a mix of all the tocopherols.

- **B-complex** helps prevent cracked lips and skin dryness and helps reduce stress.

- **Carotenoids** (precursors to vitamin A and non-toxic) keep the skin cells lying smoothly and protect against sunburn and sun damage to DNA.

- **Essential fatty acids**—omega-3 and lecithin—keep your skin smooth and supple, improve the health of your hair and nails, and help with eczema.

- **Probiotics** balance the good bacteria in the gut and help some people with rosacea, eczema, and some forms of acne.

- Liver-cleansing nutrients like **milk thistle, schisandra, and turmeric** can help with skin tone, acne, and a healthier-looking skin color.

- **Zinc** promotes growth of healthy new cells, speeds healing, helps prevent rough skin, and helps heal acne.

You can find more skin-care recommendations at my website, www.joanlubar.com.

3. Sorry, But Everyone Slows Down

No matter what, an eighty-year-old is not going to beat a forty-year-old in track and field, soccer, or dance. We just aren't built that way. Now, that forty-year-old might be able to compete against a millennial, but not without a lot of effort, training, and persistence.

However, like my seventy-something tennis-playing friend, you can still perform at a respectable, if not competitive pace by staying in good shape, maintaining proper nutrition and exercise, and using your experience and judgment.

When I began ballroom dance after fifteen years of doing only Jazzercise to keep in shape, I discovered muscles and posture that I never knew I had. It took a while to improve and be able to comfortably move across the floor again, and I am very pleased with my progress. Will I ever be able to do what I did twenty-five years ago when I was teaching, competing, and performing in the country-western dance arena? Even then, at almost fifty, I kept up with people ten or twenty years younger than I. Today I can't kick quite as high or twirl quite as fast, though I'm able to keep up with *most* of the young ones.

Don't give up when you slow down. Just wise up and use what you have!

4. Diminishing the "Dribble"

I saw the funniest cartoon years ago. It said, "I'm so old, I can laugh, cough, sneeze, and pee all at the same time." Yes, folks, this might be you, too!

Good old-fashioned Kegel exercises help both men and women. If you've forgotten how to do this, there are some excellent sites on the internet that show you easy exercises to help you find and strengthen your pelvic floor muscles. The exercises are easy and really do help! I can vouch for that.

I have been told that Pilates offers some excellent exercises for the pelvic floor that also help other muscle groups as well. I haven't tried it yet, but after researching for this chapter, I have it on my list! I know several women who swear by it, including a fifty-eight-year-old ballroom dance instructor who has the body of a thirty-year-old. She teaches Pilates and uses nutrition to stay young. For some useful information on both Kegel exercises and Pilates, check out www.verywell.com.

I have seen, but never used, a product called Intimate Rose that helps you build up your pelvic floor muscles using Kegel movements. If dribbling is more than a minor issue for you, give it a try. If the problem persists, be sure to check with your physician. In the meantime, thin panty liners are an aging woman's best friend.

Sassy Sage Dribbler's Dos and Don'ts

- Cut back on caffeine drinks and soda.

- Don't smoke.

- Keep your weight down.

- Learn pelvic floor exercises like Kegel and Pilates specific for this.

- Practice "double voiding" when you urinate. Go, relax, and then try going again.

- Keep a diary of symptoms and what you did before the leaks happened so you will have history to share with your doctor, if necessary.

A word of caution: sometimes dribbling is a symptom of a more serious medical issue, so get checked by your health professional to be sure. Good luck!

5. Almost Forgot... to Mention Memory Loss

As I completed this chapter, I wondered what I'd left out. I had to go back to the beginning to see what I'd written just a few minutes before! Yes, our memories may get a little worse and we might repeat a story yet again because we didn't remember sharing it, but we had the same lapses when we were younger, too. Think back—haven't you forgotten someone's name even when you were twenty?

When I complete a task I often feel I can drop it into some memory file and move on, sure I won't need it again. Wrong! So often I can't retrieve it from some hidden brain location, much like saving a computer file and then not knowing where it is hiding on the computer when you need it! I believe we learn SO much over the years that our brain files simply get too full. Do not despair! There are several ways to mind your memory.

Play with memorization. I once saw a man on TV who provided a trick for remembering things. When you need to remember a list of items, make funny pictures out of it and then you only have to remember the pictures. Today I remember much of that list, which included a chicken sitting on top of a bank tower, because I had to go to the bank and also buy chicken for dinner.

Puzzle power. Do you do crossword puzzles or play cards, chess, or Scrabble®? All these—and any type of puzzle—can help keep your brain working. Check out www.puzzlearttherapy.com for an integrated, holistic system that helps build and strengthen perceptual learning and sensory and creativity skills through whole-brain learning programs. Brain education through Brain & Body Yoga is also beneficial. All of these are fun, too!

Nourish your brain. Many are deficient in nutrients that feed the brain and help neurotransmitters. I already mentioned Vivix for joint pain and healing. It also helps repair DNA, keeps brain cells (and other cells) clean of debris, and helps the energy packs, or mitochondria, in our cells regenerate. Let's keep those brain cells firing on all cylinders! I also take ginkgo and ginseng for brain function.

Tend to your telomeres. Never heard of telomeres? They are the tail ends of your chromosomes, and are said to influence the rate of cellular aging: the longer, the better. One study observed a group of people who had used high-quality supplements for many years and whose telomeres had maintained their length even into their later years. The results showed that an eighty-year-old can have telomeres of the same length as a forty-year-old. The participants also had healthy diets, proper exercise, worked on stress management, and maintained a supportive social network.[9]

6. Of course, the final and truly inevitable event is death.

We can look at this in many ways, but first let's talk about preparation. Avoiding the inevitable can lead to anxiety and worry, especially for your family. Many resources are now available to help you and your family create a plan for your death, and I absolutely encourage you to do so before anything drastic happens.

When our kids were young, we were in charge. But in our older years, many of us become the children to our adult children. So while you are still feeling good and all your faculties are intact, sit down and have a peer-to-peer conversation with your kids or spouse. You will be happy you did. An excellent book I recommend is *Between You and Me* by Ali Davidson. She provides a way to have a comfortable conversation, and it is a great, respectful way to plan ahead.

---

[9] https://www.reference.com/science/happens-lengthen-telomeres-efd8bcc7ea07e21e?qo=cdpArticles

When my mom died a few years ago, I was so relieved that she was totally prepared. Her will was done, she had a trust, she had healthcare plans that insured she wouldn't have to live with (or be a burden to) any of us. She had also resolved all "old business" with my brother, sister, and me. We were all fortunate that she had taken good care of herself as well, so her passing was quick and easy. She felt she had completed her work here and kept telling me she was getting bored. One evening after dinner, she sat down, took a breath, said, "I'm dying," and at the age of ninety-six passed away peacefully. What a way to go!

My goal is to take good enough care of myself and live life fully enough so that I will come to the end as though I am sliding into home plate with a big cheer. I will have truly lived fully and had a great life! What a way to go!

You can maintain your youthfulness, no matter your age, if you make good choices, work on your attitude, rely on your support systems, and move. I can't stress it enough. While some parts of aging are indeed inevitable, being in pain, feeling bad, and looking tired and elderly are not. They are most often the result of your earlier choices. The sooner you begin to take great care of yourself, the better long-term results you'll see and feel. Invest in yourself—the return on that investment is priceless.

Accept what you cannot change, and improve what you can. Then go out and have a hell of a good time!

CHAPTER 9

YOU'RE A SPIRITUAL BEING HAVING A HUMAN EXPERIENCE

"This Magic Moment"

And then it happened
It took me by surprise
I knew that you felt it too
By the look in your eyes

This magic moment…
Will last forever
Forever till the end of time

— Ben E. King

When I was in eighth grade my science teacher taught us that everything is either energy or matter, and neither can be created or destroyed, but they are interchangeable. As we walked out of class I said to my friend, "We have been here a long time!"

That day marked the beginning of my spiritual journey. I became a seeker — devouring books and attending talks and searching for the reason why I am here.

What about you? Do you believe there is something beyond yourself? Do you spend any time reflecting on this? Many of us take so much time attending to our physical or "meat" body, or completing or worrying about all the tasks on our lists, that we forget we also have an *energy* body and a spiritual center. We forget that we have a soul.

I believe we are part of one Creator that wanted to experience more than Itself and split into millions of infinitesimal parts (including us) all having the same creative powers. And I believe that some of us realize we are part of that bigger, universal whole. By allowing us to use our creative powers (our "free will"), the Creator can experience Itself even more. We have complete free will, and yet we can always ask for help, explanations, and assistance when we need it. This Higher Power, after all, is connected to all of us, so we can go to it for any help needed. Seeking that help might look like prayer, meditation, time in nature, or any of a plethora of spiritual practices.

What this also means is that we create our own realities. We attract exactly what we need to experience in order to grow, whether we like or not. No matter what's happening in our lives, we always have the opportunity to ask ourselves, "What can I learn from this?" When we don't get the results we wanted, or when we feel like we're too old or not good enough, we can ask, "How can I make it better or move beyond this?" Sometimes we have to repeat lessons we didn't learn the first time around. And sometimes we receive a moment of grace, experiencing great joy. Whichever it is, we have brought it to us.

Have you ever met someone who has been through a horrific disease or terrible experience, and once healed, has stepped into a new and better way of being? (I know — couldn't they have found another way to learn that lesson?) You have an opportunity to do that with everything that happens to you, too.

Amy Purdy, the amazing Paralympic snowboarder, had a horrific disease that almost killed her at age eighteen, and had to have both legs amputated. That could have been the end of a full life, but instead she came back, got prosthetic legs, and began to snowboard again. She went on to get snowboarding into the Paralympics, which was a hard-fought battle, and to write her story and become a wonderful inspirational speaker.

On a smaller scale, years ago I was in a car accident. I had stopped at a light on a rainy day, just inches from the car in front. Then the car behind slammed into me and the car behind that one crashed into both of us. I felt a huge jolt from the two cars, followed by my back and neck tightening. Luckily that was the extent of my injuries.

The first thought that came to my mind was, "Why in the world did this happen to me today?" My self-response was quick: "You need to slow down and stop running around so much." Maybe that seems like a strange reaction, but I truly believe that what happens to us and what we see around us are usually signs for us to recognize and messages we need to receive. Staying distracted and stressed means we don't slow down enough to notice those signs and messages, and we miss them. I tend to slip back into that pattern of being super-busy. To this day, however, I think of that accident, and it reminds me to pull back as necessary, slow down, and rethink my schedule.

And to take my spiritual journey inside. I take time every day to be quiet in a busy, chaotic world; to go inside to my very core and hear the messages that remind me why I am here and what my real purpose is. It's my time to reconnect with my Higher Self, God, Allah, Creator—whatever name you choose. This daily reconnection brings me to an elevated state of awareness and I remember that we are all one, whatever our beliefs; that one day we really can live in harmony—with others as well as with ourselves. Sound like "pie in the sky" thinking? Maybe. But it certainly is better to me than the drama, guilt, anger, prejudice, and pathos we see around us.

Sharon O'Hara, my spiritual teacher for over thirty years, says this:

It is time for you to begin to understand and appreciate the depths and detail to which you create your own reality. Without this knowledge, you will be plagued with unforeseen (good and/or bad) situations, and believe that you are at the mercy of the situation. It is time for you to understand how you energetically attract to your experiences that can be traced...from this reality...When you look at your life, you are looking at the face of a multifaceted being put here to understand the workings of energetic fields, the movement of the celestial, and the wonders of the universe. God does not gather any praise or blemish by the good or bad done by the individuals in this world. God-Creation is only a witness to all that goes on.

We are responsible for what we think and do—and we are here for specific and unique purposes. Let's take a look at why we are here in the first place. Imagine you are a young child in the most loving family and most supportive community. Your brothers and sisters encourage you and share their knowledge; your parents nurture and love you; your neighbors always look out for you; and your teachers help you learn in the most positive ways.

You have gone from kindergarten through twelfth grade and it is now time to prepare for college. You sit with your counselor to discuss the curriculum you will be taking. You pick your courses: parents, siblings, career, location, health, and intelligence, and you even pick your own personal assignment and your greater purpose, that thing you are to learn for yourself. Now you are ready to go to the college of your choice: Planet Earth.

You always have assistance. Some of us call these angels or guides. I prefer "Soul Friends"—spirits similar to us who are just not in human form. Right up until your entrance into the birth canal, they are there, so if you choose not to move into a human life, they can help you return to that loving world. They then step away for your birth, and during that time you forget all that you have planned and set in place. You are now on Earth and your job is to "re-member" why you are here.

While this may seem far-fetched, doesn't it make sense that we have all come here with some type of plan? Some purpose to fulfill? Otherwise why would one child be born to abusive parents while another is born to a loving family that supports them in every way; or one child is born completely healthy and the next has cerebral palsy or is disfigured? What have they chosen to learn and how long do they choose to be here to work on it?

Please do not think that because I hold this view I am not appalled at some of the tragedy and ugliness I have seen. The difference is perspective: What lesson can we learn from this? How does it play into our moving forward to live more purpose-driven lives, however small or large, and to make a difference in our communities?

I believe that my path is in front of me and that my choices, for which I am responsible, either good or bad, will lead me to fulfill my reason for being here. Of course, getting some higher awareness and consciousness along the way certainly helps! Then, when I have completed my purpose, it will be time to go—or perhaps I will even get to choose to hang out a little longer and just play! Either way, we each have our own story to create, and we might want to step back and make sure we are not taking on someone else's instead.

Have you ever noticed that a reaction you have to something might not be yours? The story I told earlier in which I gave back to my son his response to something I was accused of is an example. Many of us have taken on beliefs of our parents, teachers, or communities without ever stepping back to discover what we truly believe in our hearts.

Do you remember the movie *Made in Heaven*? In it, Timothy Hutton plays a young man who dies trying to keep a family from drowning in a river. He then falls in love with one of the souls he meets in Heaven. She gets called to come to Earth, and he begs to also be returned. He is given thirty years to find her. On his thirtieth birthday, after having just missed her several times but never connecting, they finally get together. I love the movie because it speaks to that notion that we come to Earth with a certain mission.

The point is that we all have the chance to fulfill our plans and live lives that are meaningful and purposeful. Being aware that we have this choice, though, can really help us get on track more quickly.

In my life I've navigated an unbelievable number of transitions, open doors, closed doors, and learning experiences (another word for "challenges"), but because I learned over thirty years ago that I am more than this body, I have been able to work my way through, grow from the experiences, and reach a higher level of awareness than I ever thought possible.

Years ago I was in a small town in India called Yogaville that was founded by a swami. In the Lotus Temple there, was a room with altars for all known religions — those that are no longer here and those yet to be. Above them was a sign that said, "The Truth is one; the Paths are many." That made so much sense to me. When we were introduced to the swami, I saw in his sparkling blue eyes a depth of peace, love, and contentment. I felt taken to another level of love and joy in that short meeting. He was truly in the state of oneness I have been describing — it's what I personally desire to reach.

Whatever your belief system, you can become more aware and closer to that feeling of oneness. My dear friend Helen is a ninety-three-year-old devout Catholic who prays several times a day and feels comfort and peace as she connects with Mother Mary. It is clear to me that she reaches those realms of "oneness" even if she would never define it that way.

Another thing that keeps my energy high is that I don't judge what others believe. Unless they are trying to harm others, everyone is free to connect, worship, and believe as they choose. I don't believe that anyone has the right to tell me what I should or should not believe even if I ask for their opinion. I believe that is why I chose to be born in the US, even though we still have a way to go in living the truth of this fundamental concept of our Bill of Rights.

How do my spiritual beliefs keep me feeling young and healthy?

When I first moved to Oregon, I remember driving along I-84 and gasping as I saw the magnificence of Mount Hood soaring above everything else in the distance. I was overcome with a sense of awe at how small we are in comparison — and how filled with possibility seeing that mountain made me feel. The same is true in reaching higher levels of consciousness, learning that while we are small, we also have the whole universe and cosmos within us. Just as I described in regard to our mental attitudes, we actually physically and hormonally feel better and look younger when we allow ourselves to be part of something greater than ourselves.

We all function better when we remember that we are more than just our bodies. And when that realization happens, we can't help but become kinder, less angry, and more forgiving. On the spiritual level, we grow closer to our true selves — the souls or spirits that are our essences. On the physical level, we produce more serotonin, which in turn makes us happier and look and feel younger.

How do you reach this state of awareness, especially if you have way too much on your plate and are angry at the world (or one particular person)? And what if you are suffering from a major disease or grieving the death of a close friend or family member? My other strategies deal with well-being and mental/emotional state. I am now talking about strategies that help you connect with your inner self, your soul, and the "All That Is." The way to do this is to carve out some quiet time. Here are some of the pieces of my spiritual practice:

1. **Breathe.** Begin by breathing deeply from your diaphragm. You do this naturally when you lie down, so try it and see how it feels. Breathe in through your nose to the count of four, hold for four, and then breathe out through your mouth for eight counts. When particularly stressed, I breathe in and think "I am" and breathe out "peace." It feels so good! Just do it until you calm down.

2. **Take a yoga class**, especially if you are in a constant state of physical stress that is showing up in tight muscles, headaches, or tension in your belly.

3. **Read a book** about connecting with your Higher Self. I love literature that reminds me that you and I are more than just our bodies. One book I often recommend is *Awakening the Spirit Within* by Rebecca Rosen.

4. Take a few minutes each day to **reconnect with your Higher Self** (or whatever you call who created you) **through prayer or meditation**. Your goal is to remember that you are so much more than the meat body. If you can carve out a specific time daily, even five minutes at first, this is your way to remind yourself who you really are.

a. Put your focus above your head and feel the divine light or gold sparkles coming through the top of your head, down your spine, and through your body. If you are familiar with the chakra system, send this light through each chakra.

b. **Create positive affirmation(s)** that speak to who you are or want to become, and use this time to repeat them to yourself. Think things like "I am_____." You can choose anything that helps you create a better life or self-perspective. "I am" kind, loving, helpful, successful, powerful.

c. You can also say "I choose_____," perhaps to help you make decisions that create a more positive, fulfilling life.

5. **Rely more on your intuition.** This is the closest you come to messages from your Higher Self. We are not talking emotional decisions, but what comes in during a quiet moment of deliberation. Trust yourself. Ask for what you need. Pay attention to the signs and messages you receive.

6. **Be grateful.** Yes, this again! Each day for thirty days, write down five things you are grateful for, adding "Thank you, thank you, thank you" at the end of each. Then take time each morning or evening to note what you are grateful for that day. These can be small things or major events.

7. **Forgive yourself.** Everyone is always doing the best they can at any given moment, even if it is not the best they are capable of. That is a big concept to swallow, especially with all of the meanness and violence we see daily. But start with yourself. Your essence is part of the One; you are perfect. We often let the layers of our upbringings and our environments take over, and make choices that are not the best. Self-forgiveness reminds us that we can move forward and create better lives and a better world.

We have always been led, are being led, and, if we allow it, will always be led. We just need to open up to all of the messages. I want to share a quote from Neale Donald Walsch, author of *Conversations with God*, from one of his "Daily Inspiration" emails:

… all of life is animated by a single fantastic energy,
which is the essence of everything that is—including you.
Isn't that amazing? Now, because this essence is who
you are and what you are made of, it can obviously
never leave you.
Perhaps not so obviously, it can also be wonderfully helpful.
It can bring you peace in moments of stress,
Strength in moments of weakness
Courage in moments of fear,
Wisdom in moments of confusion,
Forgiveness in moments of anger
And love in all the moments of your life.
All you have to do is know that this is true,
And it will be true for you, right now.

CHAPTER 10

PUTTING IT ALL TOGETHER

"Imagine"

You may say I'm a dreamer
But I'm not the only one
I hope someday you'll join us
And the world will be as one

— John Lennon

Thank you for going on this journey with me! I hope *Rock and Roll at Any Age* has given you some ideas and insights about staying youthful and healthy no matter what your age. And I hope it's also inspired you to turn on some good ol' rock-and-roll and dance around your living room.

I have an image to leave you with. Think of your physical body as a car—the only car you will have in this lifetime. Think about how you would take care of that vehicle so it lasts as long as you do. Here is some of the maintenance that would need to be done:

- Change the oil regularly
- Check all fluids in a timely manner and keep them at the correct levels

- Check and replace brakes, as necessary
- Keep the car clean
- Schedule regular checkups to ensure all is working well
- Immediately handle unexpected problems

As with a car, you can get by with some minor symptoms for a while, but eventually, if you don't get to the cause, you'll have a breakdown.

A few months ago a triangular light with an exclamation point kept showing up on my dash. This happened off and on so I stopped by my mechanic to see what it was. I thought it was the tire pressure since it began after I had two new tires put on, so he checked it. He said everything looked fine and told me to bring it back if the light continued.

One morning I set out for a meeting in a city a few hours away. The light now was on almost constantly, so when I saw a truck stop, I followed my intuition to stop there and get a second opinion. What happened next made me keenly aware that if something seems amiss, it probably is, and I should get to the bottom of it before a major incident happens.

I was down to less than a quart of oil! Had I continued on I would have been in deep trouble. When your car doesn't have enough oil it doesn't benefit from oil's normal function — cleaning, lubricating, and cooling your engine system — and will start to build up tar, sludge, and soot. Your whole system will suffer wear and tear at a faster rate.

Needless to say, I added nearly five quarts of oil and continued my trip. When I got home I had the whole system checked.

We all have little complaints, sometimes on a daily basis, that we think of as aging or some other excuse. These symptoms are your body talking to you, just like that triangular light was talking to me. You can just let them go or you can make an effort to determine what is going on.

Do you have a nutritional deficiency?

Are you under a lot of stress, which depletes your body in so many ways?

Do you have a virus or bacterial infection?

As I noted earlier, when something's going on with my body, I always look at what is happening in my life emotionally and what my current eating habits are. I then check the symptoms against what deficiencies can cause them, and tune in to what my current stress level and attitude are. I always prefer a natural approach, knowing the body can heal itself, but if necessary I go to my healthcare professional for more extensive crisis care. (I certainly wouldn't expect a multivitamin to fix a broken leg!)

You can keep your body going by making good choices. By remaining youthful and vibrant you can be more of a contribution to our world. The one-car-per-life image addresses the physical body, but without a driver to turn it on, the car is useless. How you drive the car is determined by your mindset at any given moment. Do everything you can to keep your attitude positive, and always remember that you are so much more than your physical body. Remembering both can help you prevent reckless and careless driving and help avoid the "accidents" of life choices. Your thoughts direct where your energy goes, creating the reality you choose to live.

Tending to Our Society

For years now the emphasis has been on youth—expensive, dangerous surgery to look younger; listening only to young people; pushing older, experienced workers out of the culture and the workforce; and ignoring the ideas and wisdom of elders in the family. Do you realize what society is missing? Have you, if you are older, realized that you have bought into this attitude?

As we age, it's our time to join ranks and stand up to be heard and appreciated for our value. When society ignores its older citizens' knowledge, experience, and wisdom, it has fallen prey to the brashness and arrogance of many younger leaders who have decided they know all the answers. It has also created a generation that ignores and disrespects the older generation. Perhaps older people were that way when they were young, too.

In our older years most of us have learned to be more patient and to listen more closely and then decide what we can offer. Our younger friends have no idea what they are missing—they haven't been there yet!

I see many people my age and older who have given up. Many sit and watch TV all day, wondering what has happened. I encourage all of us, young and old, to look for ways to create more community, connection, and cooperation. If you are young, just reach out and listen. Imagine the amazing stories and wisdom and life experiences you might hear; you can then make your own decisions about life with a whole new perspective. If you are older, accept that young people might not agree with you, but that at least you can offer your opinions based on your interactions and experience. Life is about building quality relationships, and often elders are treated as the invisible ones who have no value.

Not true!! As Baby Boomers reach the age of seniors, they are crying out, "Wait a minute! I am still a valuable asset to society and family! Don't throw me away!" I encourage all who are reading this book to take a new look. We can age and be productive. We can give back by helping mentor our younger folks, by participating in community activities, and by raising our voices together, not separately.

My final wish for you is that you become a rock star in your own life! Get up and rock and roll! Take yourself and your choices seriously, and then get out into the world and become the person you are meant to be, no matter what your age.

Life is to be enjoyed, not endured.

We all deserve it!

RESOURCES

Here are the resources I've noted throughout the book, plus links for much of the information I provided. Please connect with me if you have any questions at joan@joanlubar.com. It has been a pleasure sharing this book and these ideas with you!

1. Dr. Christiane Northrup: I just love her video at http://bit.ly/DrNorthrup-V2. While it is part of a series, it is also a great overview of how we are not aging but making choices that we attribute to aging, plus three amazing exercises to do daily. Along with my three-minute exercise program, you can see a major difference within two weeks!

2. How Do You Feel? Questionnaire

HOW DO YOU FEEL?

Many of us have little aches, pains, and annoying concerns for which we don't go for medical help. These symptoms may have larger implications or be precursors of something major down the road. Often by making some small changes you can minimize or eliminate these minor concerns and avoid long-term consequences.

Below are some of those symptoms that you might consider unimportant. Your body is asking you for some help, so start listening to it.

Please mark the blank to the left of each symptom as follows:

1 = mild 2 = moderate 3 = severe

___No pep

___Overweight/Underweight

___Splitting, breaking fingernails

___Dull, thinning hair

___Need coffee, tea, soda to keep going

___Headaches/Migraines

___Great desire for chocolate, sweets

___Constipation, hemorrhoids

___Bleeding gums

___Bruise easily

___Take aspirin, Tylenol, Advil often

___Poor digestion

___Poor circulation/cold hands and feet

___Hard to wake up/get up in morning

___Can't fall asleep or stay asleep

___Dry/oily skin

___Complexion problems

___Leg cramps

___Bad breath/Smelly feet

___Subject to colds and infections

___Nervous or depressed

___Various aches and pains

___Have vague "blah" feeling

___Require tranquilizers

___Use antacids

___Shortness of breath

___Under stress

___High cholesterol/triglycerides

___Sinus and allergy problems

___Backaches

___Joint stiffness

___Water retention

___Menstrual cramps/PMS

___Hot flashes

___Psoriasis

What is the most important challenge you have with your health or your family's health?

How long has this been going on?

What have you done about it?

On a scale of 1-10, how well has it worked?

If you could change just one thing about your or your family's health, what would it be?

Would you like a free analysis and recommendations? Email this questionnaire to joan@joanlubar.com

NAME: _____ PHONE: _____

3. What product lines do I recommend?

Supplement companies and the herbal industry are very poorly (if at all) regulated. Here is a list of things to ask or research about brands. (Thank you, Dr. Bruce Miller.)

a. Are the products backed by published clinical research studies?

b. Are the health and nutrient claims, if any, based on anecdotal information or on scientific data?

c. Do they have peer-reviewed published research?

d. What information is available on ingredient specifications, safety, and quality testing?

e. Is there published evidence of their products' absorption into the bloodstream (bioavailability)?

f. What proof do they have of product stability? For example, product testing on a group of probiotics showed that none to one-third of live bacteria in the products reached the small intestine; the rest died. And 39 out of 43 ginseng products contained no active ingredients.

g. Do they test for contaminants and heavy metals such as lead, cadmium, arsenic, etc.? Many supplement companies do not.

h. Do they have proven research that their products have been clinically tested, preferably published in peer-reviewed journals such as the *Journal of Clinical Nutrition*, the *American Journal of Cardiology*, the *Journal of Applied Physiology*, or the *Journal of the American College of Nutrition*?

I choose Shaklee Corporation's products and have used them for over thirty years because they match the above criteria and are tested for purity all the way through the manufacturing process with guaranteed results. I use their skin-care products, too, which contain pure ingredients and nutrients that enhance the skin and help prevent aging. Like the supplements, they are clinically tested and researched for effectiveness and quality. See more information at http://shaklee.tv/enfuselle-from-shaklee. To purchase go to https://jlahealthstop.myshaklee.com/us/en/shop/healthybeauty. Other companies that seem to have quality programs and research:

Life Extension: I have not used their products, but their articles and research look good.

Usana: A well-respected company whose products have very good research and testing.

Personal Care Products: Do not have a long list of toxic chemicals in their products, and they can prove it.

Beauty Counter: They produce cosmetics that contain pure ingredients, eliminating over 1,500 potentially toxic ingredients. For more information, check out www.beautycounter.com/EmilyGuerrero.

Green Cleaners:

Shaklee's line of cleaners, dishwashing, and laundry products are green, effective, and economical. They carry disinfectants, general cleaning products, deodorizers, degreasers, presoaks, and more, and they're easy to use. For more information, go to https://jlahealthstop.myshaklee.com/us/en/shop/healthyhome.

Other product lines I recommend include Mrs. Meyers Clean Day, Seventh Generation, and Maleleuca.

Enjo's products contain specially designed fibers that work with just water (and with other green cleaners). The link for their products is www.emilyguerrero.ezgreenclean.com.

Lemon, baking soda, and vinegar: Different combinations of these items work on everything from showers to toilets.

Food Supplement Programs:

My beginning program includes:

- a protein shake
- a multivitamin/mineral
- Shaklee Herb-Lax (the first laxative I tried that was gentle, worked for me, and helped normalize the blood — a signature Dr. Shaklee product)

My mid-level foundational program includes:

Cleansing:

alfalfa

Herb-Lax

probiotics (I use Shaklee Optiflora Probiotic Complex® if I'm not also using a protein drink that contains live bacteria.)

Cell and immune builders:

> Shaklee Life Plan protein shakes, which are also meal replacements, include omega-3s, prebiotics, and probiotics that don't die in stomach acid.
> Shaklee Vita Lea® multivitamin/mineral
> extra vitamin C (Shaklee Vita C® Sustained-release, because it spreads out over five hours)
> extra B-complex for stress and nerves

Now I use a high-level foundational program that includes:

Cleansing: same as above

Cell and immune builders:

> Shaklee Life Plan protein shakes
> Shaklee Vitalizer™, a bubble strip of doses that contain all the vitamins listed for the mid-level program above plus extra antioxidants, vitamin E, and omega-3 fish oil

4. Resetting My Metabolism: I love the easy five-day reset program below for resetting your metabolism and getting you back on track when you've strayed from a healthy diet. It is especially good at holiday time in between parties and temptations. It is also a great way to start a weight-management or weight-loss program because it minimizes cravings for sweets and simple carbs.

5 Day Reset Plan

Increase Energy, Lose Weight, Reset Metabolism

Wake-Up:

- Drink detox tea (30 minutes before eating breakfast if you can)

- 16 oz. water (hot, cold, or room temperature)
- 1/2 squeezed lemon or lime
- Shaklee 180® Energy Tea, any flavor

Optional: 1 scoop of Shaklee Performance®

Breakfast:
- Shaklee Life smoothie
- 5 Shaklee Alfalfa Complex
- 1 to 4 Shaklee Liver DTX® Complex (begin with one, then add a second, etc.)

Optional: Shaklee Vitalizer™ or Life-Strip

Snack choices:
- Unlimited organic raw veggies
- Shaklee 180® Snack Bar
- Hummus
- Hard-boiled egg

Lunch:
- Shaklee Life smoothie and/or organic salad

Snack choices:
- Shaklee 180® Snack Bar
- Unlimited organic raw veggies
- hummus
- fruit

Dinner:
- Shaklee Life smoothie
– organic salad
– 5 Shaklee Alfalfa Complex
- 2 Shaklee Liver DTX Complex
- 2 Shaklee Herb-Lax

Lemon water all day:

1/2 oz. water per pound of body weight (150 pound person = 75 ounces lemon water)

5. Women's Health: While a more thorough assessment is worthwhile, here are a couple of tips from my experiences:

PMS and/or Cramps: Add calcium to your diet or supplements during the month, and an even greater amount two to four days before you expect your period to start. I recommend OsteoMatrix® by Shaklee because it includes all the nutrients that help absorb the calcium better.

Irritability: Add extra vitamin B-complex to your diet or supplements daily, and an even greater amount two to four days before you expect your period to start. This helps with hormone balance as well. I recommend Shaklee B-Complex for a pure, well-balanced vitamin B combination.

Perimenopause: For some, additional vitamin E helps with symptoms. It should, however, be natural and a combination of mixed tocopherols. Again, I depend on Shaklee's Vita-E Complex®.

Menopause: There are several herbs that help relieve symptoms, including several Chinese herbs and certain essential oils. I recommend a combination of black cohosh, don quai, red clover, soy isoflavones, and flaxseed oil. Menopause Balance Complex® by Shaklee is a good choice.

A complete article on women's hormonal imbalances can be found at my website, www.joanlubar.com, under "Articles/Videos."

6. Candida albicans revisited: Excess yeast in your system can be an underlying cause of many diseases. Below are some sources:

Dr. Eric Bakker, at www.ericbakker.com, provides extensive information, some of which you read about above.

Dr. Josh Axe, at www.draxe.com, also has excellent information, some of which I provide below. The complete article is available at https://draxe.com/candida-symptoms. He lists these symptoms:

- Exhaustion
- Cravings for sweets
- Bad breath
- White coat on tongue (oral thrush)
- Brain fog
- Mood disorders
- Hormone imbalance
- Joint pain
- Loss of sex drive
- Chronic sinus and allergy issues
- Digestive problems (gas and bloating)
- Weak immune system
- Vaginal and/or urinary tract infections

"Candida Overgrowth Syndrome, or COS, is the term used when candida has grown out of control in your body. Make no mistake; this is a chronic health condition. Individuals… can find they have developed new sensitivities, allergies or intolerances to a variety of foods. These foods include dairy, eggs, corn and gluten."

Some causes of candida infections:

- Broad-spectrum antibiotics
- Birth control pills
- Oral corticosteroids
- Cancer treatments
- Diabetes
- Weakened immune system

Some of Dr. Axe's recommendations are:

- Coconut oil, through both ingestion and as a topical application
- Milk thistle [from Joan: Shaklee's Liver DTX® Complex has milk thistle and others herbs that support this, and is well researched and tested for potency.]
- Vitamin C
- Clove oil, oregano oil, and myrrh essential oils

"Candida die-off symptoms you may experience:

- Impaired brain function
- Headache
- Fatigue

- Dizziness
- Intestinal distress including bloating, gas, constipation, nausea
- Sweating and fever
- Sinus infection
- Skin breakouts (not limited to face)
- Typical flu-like symptoms
- Typically clears up in 7 to 10 days"

Both Dr. Bakker and Dr. Axe recommend programs for overcoming candida. I recommend reading both websites to find an option that is comfortable for you. You are also welcome to contact me to discuss it.

7. Sugar Choices

We have all heard about how bad sugar is for us. When eaten in whole foods, however, sugar content is balanced by fiber, making absorption take longer and avoiding sugar spikes, which are so damaging to our health. Using the information below about **glycemic index and glycemic load** as they relate to sugar intake will help you make good choices. Your choices can affect weight loss, weight gain, and the increased possibility of diabetes and cardiovascular problems.

The **glycemic index (GI)** provides a measure of how quickly blood glucose (sugar) level rises after a particular food is eaten. The effects that different foods have on blood glucose level can vary considerably. This index estimates how much each gram of available carbohydrate (total carbohydrate minus fiber) in a food raises a person's blood glucose level following the consumption of the food, relative to the consumption of pure glucose. Glucose has a GI of 100.[10] The number can vary due to ripeness, preparation, and storage methods, but still provides a good baseline. Above 55 is considered high, but a key is the glycemic load number—see below.

The **glycemic load (GL)** of food is a number that estimates how much the food raises a person's blood glucose level after eating it. One unit of GL approximates the effect of consuming one gram of glucose. GL accounts for how much carbohydrate is in the food and how much each gram of carbohydrate in the food raises blood glucose. GL is based on GI, and is calculated by multiplying the grams of available carbohydrate in the food times the food's GI, and then dividing by 100. For one serving of a food, **a GL greater than 20 is considered high, a GL of 11 to 19 is considered medium, and a GL of 10 or less is considered low.** Foods that have a low GL in a typical serving size almost always have a low GI. Foods with an intermediate or high GL in a typical serving size range from a very low to a very high GI. GL seems to be an important factor in insulin resistance, metabolic syndrome, and weight loss.[11]

---

[10] https://ultimatepaleoguide.com/glycemic-index-food-list

[11] http://www.wikipedia.org

Glycemic Index & Glycemic Load Index For 100+ Foods[12]

FOOD	Glycemic index (glucose = 100)	Serving size (grams)	Glycemic load per serving
BAKERY PRODUCTS AND BREADS			
Banana cake, made with sugar	47	60	14
Banana cake, made without sugar	55	60	12
Sponge cake, plain	46	63	17
Vanilla cake made from packet mix with vanilla frosting (Betty Crocker)	42	111	24
Apple, made with sugar	44	60	13
Apple, made without sugar	48	60	9
Waffles, Aunt Jemima (Quaker Oats)	76	35	10
Bagel, white, frozen	72	70	25
Baguette, white, plain	95	30	15
Coarse barley bread, 75-80% kernels, average	34	30	7
Hamburger bun	61	30	9
Kaiser roll	73	30	12
Pumpernickel bread	56	30	7
50% cracked wheat kernel bread	58	30	12
White wheat flour bread	71	30	10
Wonder™ bread, average	73	30	10
Whole wheat bread, average	71	30	9
100% Whole Grain™ bread (Natural Ovens)	51	30	7

Pita bread, white	68	30	10
Corn tortilla	52	50	12
Wheat tortilla	30	50	8
BEVERAGES			
Coca Cola®, average	63	250 mL	16
Fanta®, orange soft drink	68	250 mL	23
Lucozade®, original (sparkling glucose drink)	95±10	250 mL	40
Apple juice, unsweetened, average	44	250 mL	30
Cranberry juice cocktail (Ocean Spray®)	68	250 mL	24
Gatorade	78	250 mL	12
Orange juice, unsweetened	50	250 mL	12
Tomato juice, canned	38	250 mL	4
BREAKFAST CEREALS AND RELATED PRODUCTS			
All-Bran™, average	55	30	12
Coco Pops™, average	77	30	20
Cornflakes™, average	93	30	23
Cream of Wheat™ (Nabisco)	66	250	17
Cream of Wheat™, Instant (Nabisco)	74	250	22
Grape-Nuts™, average	75	30	16
Muesli, average	66	30	16
Oatmeal, average	55	250	13
Instant oatmeal, average	83	250	30
Puffed wheat, average	80	30	17
Raisin Bran™ (Kellogg's)	61	30	12
Special K™ (Kellogg's)	69	30	14

GRAINS			
Pearled barley, average	28	150	12
Sweet corn on the cob, average	60	150	20
Couscous, average	65	150	9
Quinoa	53	150	13
White rice, average	89	150	43
Quick cooking white basmati	67	150	28
Brown rice, average	50	150	16
Converted, white rice (Uncle Ben's®)	38	150	14
Whole wheat kernels, average	30	50	11
Bulgur, average	48	150	12
COOKIES AND CRACKERS			
Graham crackers	74	25	14
Vanilla wafers	77	25	14
Shortbread	64	25	10
Rice cakes, average	82	25	17
Rye crisps, average	64	25	11
Soda crackers	74	25	12
DAIRY PRODUCTS AND ALTERNATIVES			
Ice cream, regular	57	50	6
Ice cream, premium	38	50	3
Milk, full fat	41	250mL	5
Milk, skim	32	250 mL	4
Reduced-fat yogurt with fruit, average	33	200	11
FRUITS			
Apple, average	39	120	6
Banana, ripe	62	120	16
Dates, dried	42	60	18

Grapefruit	25	120	3
Grapes, average	59	120	11
Orange, average	40	120	4
Peach, average	42	120	5
Peach, canned in light syrup	40	120	5
Pear, average	38	120	4
Pear, canned in pear juice	43	120	5
Prunes, pitted	29	60	10
Raisins	64	60	28
Watermelon	72	120	4
BEANS AND NUTS			
Baked beans, average	40	150	6
Blackeye peas, average	33	150	10
Black beans	30	150	7
Chickpeas, average	10	150	3
Chickpeas, canned in brine	38	150	9
Navy beans, average	31	150	9
Kidney beans, average	29	150	7
Lentils, average	29	150	5
Soy beans, average	15	150	1
Cashews, salted	27	50	3
Peanuts, average	7	50	0
PASTA and NOODLES			
Fettuccini, average	32	180	15
Macaroni, average	47	180	23
Macaroni and Cheese (Kraft)	64	180	32
Spaghetti, white, boiled, average	46	180	22
Spaghetti, white, boiled 20 min, average	58	180	26
Spaghetti, wholemeal, boiled, average	42	180	17

SNACK FOODS			
Corn chips, plain, salted, average	42	50	11
Fruit Roll-Ups®	99	30	24
M & M's®, peanut	33	30	6
Microwave popcorn, plain, average	55	20	6
Potato chips, average	51	50	12
Pretzels, oven-baked	83	30	16
Snickers Bar®	51	60	18
VEGETABLES			
Green peas, average	51	80	4
Carrots, average	35	80	2
Parsnips	52	80	4
Baked russet potato, average	111	150	33
Boiled white potato, average	82	150	21
Instant mashed potato, average	87	150	17
Sweet potato, average	70	150	22
Yam, average	54	150	20
MISCELLANEOUS			
Hummus (chickpea salad dip)	6	30	0
Chicken nuggets, frozen, reheated in microwave oven 5 min	46	100	7
Pizza, plain baked dough, served with parmesan cheese and tomato sauce	80	100	22
Pizza, Super Supreme (Pizza Hut)	36	100	9
Honey, average	61	25	12

[12] https://ultimatepaleoguide.com/glycemic-index-food-list

ACKNOWLEDGMENTS

What a journey this has been! There are many people to thank for helping me complete this project.

I first want to thank my mom, who is no longer with us. Whatever our times of conflict, she always supported and encouraged me and pushed me to be the best I could be. She must be up there smiling, as I have begun to do some of the things I resisted for so long!

Next is my unbelievable marketing coach and friend, Kathleen Gage. Because she kept me accountable, setting up interviews with me for each chapter, I got down to work and began to really do the work. She has a whole program to help writers get their books to market, which helped me understand all the work needed. She also held my hand as I gave her many blank stares!

I could not have completed this book without the help of Madeleine Eno, the most wonderful editor on the planet! She totally understood me and what I was trying to share and was able to clarify concepts and stories that didn't always come out quite the way I wanted to express them.

Other thank yous go to Robyn MacKillop, who has been trying to teach me how to effectively use social media (say a prayer for her); Kerry Yu of OPearl Brands (see one of her necklaces on the cover), who is helping me reach the public; and Leslie Akins, who is graphic designer extraordinaire for my cover. My angels!

Lynne Klippel of Business Building Books did the final work to get my book published, including the final copyediting and whatever else was necessary to get it to market. I felt like I was giving her my newborn and she gently held it and moved it where it was meant to be. Her staff has been incredibly helpful in getting this book published, especially editor Gwen Hoffnagle.

Thank you all for this amazing team effort that kept me on track and sane in this journey. I love you all!

ABOUT THE AUTHOR

Joan Lubar is a "recovering" CPA and contract servicing analyst who has been in the wellness business for over thirty years helping others take responsibility for their lives and their health. She started her own health and wellness business after using alternative methods to regain her own health and has done presentations and health counseling since then. She has worked with well-known nutritionists and physicians to expand her nutrition and health knowledge and has earned certifications in nutrition and wellness education.

Joan's journey in the world of complementary wellness care and taking responsibility for her own health took her from being forty and tired, falling asleep at work, and gaining weight to being a vibrant, energetic, and fun-filled senior, feeling fit and fabulous!

Life always takes its twists and turns. For Joan there have been many twists that brought her to the balanced, forward-looking woman she is today. Helping her former husband, who has Parkinson's, led her to learning about caregiving and enhanced her knowledge of improving the health of those with Parkinson's-type diseases and slowing the progression of these diseases through natural means.

One of Joan's loves is dancing, which she has done since she was five! Just put some good, rhythmic music on and you will see her begin to move! Over the years she has taught, competed, and judged in the country-western world and now enjoys ballroom dancing for fun. Her theme is "Rock around the Clock!"

Joan has a passion for helping others recognize their value, especially seniors who are often treated like they are "over the hill." In her workshops she emphasizes individual responsibility for one's health and provides solutions for making each day a vibrant, joyful one. Her mission is to help older adults stay vital and engaged as they age, feeling and looking as youthful as possible, as long as possible. They then can participate in and be reconnected with their communities as viable contributors who have experience and wisdom.

Joan Lubar
info@joanlubar.com
joanlubar.com
rockandrollatanyage.com

49662663R00094

Made in the USA
San Bernardino, CA
01 June 2017